THE
MT. SHASTA BOOK

THIRD EDITION

Praise for *The Mt. Shasta Book*

The Mt. Shasta Book *demonstrates that it's more than a straightforward guide to Shasta's skiing and trekking routes . . . Selters and Zanger offer sound advice on avoiding hazards while never sounding preachy. Instead, they give the common-sense approaches that will put you in touch with the strange, almost mystical beauty of the mountain while telling you the smart ways to avoid the peak when the complexities of weather or terrain make it dangerous . . . Well worth the cover price.*
—Powder Magazine

. . . an exhaustive guide to the hiking trails and climbing routes on this massive volcano... [the] map is excellent.
—The Climbing Art

At long last, Andy Selters and Mike Zanger have given hikers, climbers and skiers the key that unlocks the treasure chest that is Mt. Shasta. Buy a copy and head for the mountain.
— Nick Clinch, past President, American Alpine Club

Anyone who climbs, skis, hikes, bikes, walks or simply enjoys looking at Mt. Shasta needs a copy of The Mt. Shasta Book. It is a wealth of information and guidance, especially for those interested in some of the finest and most spectacular back country skiing in America.
— Dick Dorworth,
former U.S. Olympic Ski Coach

Lucid, luminous, well organized and informed. A real wise guide.
— Paul McHugh, *San Francisco Chronicle*

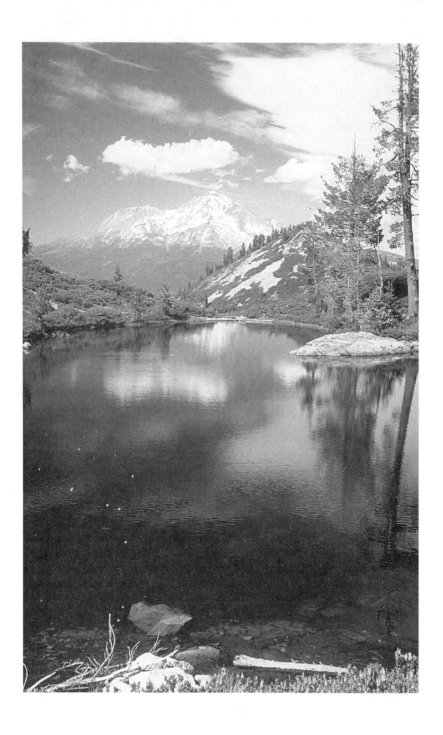

THE
MT. SHASTA BOOK

THIRD EDITION

A Guide to Hiking, Climbing, Skiing,
and Exploring the Mountain
and Surrounding Area

Andy Selters
Michael Zanger

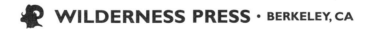 **WILDERNESS PRESS** · BERKELEY, CA

The Mt. Shasta Book

1st EDITION August 1989
2nd EDITION February 2001
3rd EDITION May 2006
  2nd printing January 2009

Copyright © 1989, 2001, 2006 by Andy Selters and Michael Zanger

Front cover photos copyright © 2006 by Andy Selters and Michael Zanger
All interior photographs by the authors, except where otherwise credited

Cover and book design: Lisa Pletka

ISBN 978-0-89997-404-0

Manufactured in the United States of America

Published by: Wilderness Press
               1345 8th Street
               Berkeley, CA 94710
               (800) 443-7227; FAX (510) 558-1696
               info@wildernesspress.com
               www.wildernesspress.com

               Visit our website for a complete listing of our books and for
               ordering information.

Cover photos: Mt. Shasta *(top);* climbers on Hotlum-Bolam Ridge
Frontispiece: Heart Lake

SAFETY NOTICE: Although Wilderness Press and the author have made
every attempt to ensure that the information in this book is accurate at press
time, they are not responsible for any loss, damage, injury, or inconvenience
that may occur to anyone while using this book. You are responsible for your
own safety and health while in the wilderness. The fact that a route is
described in this book does not mean that it will be safe for you. Be aware that
trail conditions can change from day to day. Always check local conditions and
know your own limitations.

ACKNOWLEDGMENTS

Without the help and support of many of those who love Mt. Shasta and associate themselves with the mountain, this book would have barely been possible. We would especially like to thank geologists Dan Miller, Paul Dawson and Bruce Friend, botanist Dr. William Bridge Cooke, College of the Siskiyous librarian Dennis Freeman, archaeologist and anthropologist Julie Krieger, meteorologist Jim DePree, whitewater sage John Googins, Siskiyou County Deputy Sheriff Charlie Simpson, Lee Apperson and the Sisson Hatchery Museum, aerial photo expert Egon Harrasser, Edward Stuhl, and the Bancroft Library.

Special thanks also to Chris and Jenn Carr, Nick Crane, Sean Doyle, Tom Hesseldenz, Matt Hill, Phil Holecek, Steve Johnson, Larry Jordan, Michael Kirwin, Steven Labensart, Chris Marrone, Penn Martin, Ron McDowell, Paul McHugh, Bill Miese, Jack Moore, Ken Morrish, Manny Navarro, Phil Rhodes, Mark Rodell, Perry Sims, Dan Towner, Eric White, Chris and Sierra Zanger, the "lean, young pros" at Shasta Mountain Guides, and the folks at The Fifth Season . . . all mountain people at heart.

—*Andy Selters and Michael Zanger*
Bishop & Mount Shasta
February 2006

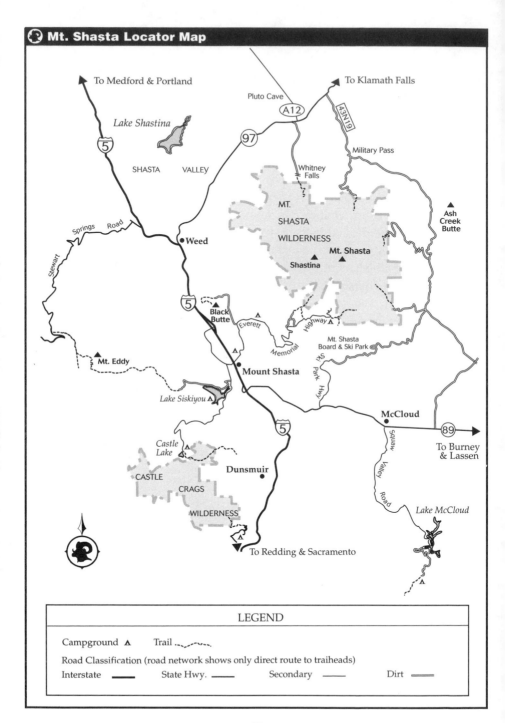

Mt. Shasta Locator Map

To Medford & Portland

Lake Shastina

Pluto Cave

To Klamath Falls

A12

43N19

97

Military Pass

SHASTA   VALLEY

Whitney
Falls

MT.

SHASTA

WILDERNESS

Ash
Creek
Butte

Springs   Road

5

•Weed

Mt. Shasta

Shastina

Stewart

5

Black
Butte

Everett

Mt. Shasta
Board & Ski Park

Mt. Eddy

Memorial

Highway

Ski Park Hwy

• Mount Shasta

Lake Siskiyou

McCloud
•

Castle
Lake

5

89

Squaw

To Burney
& Lassen

CASTLE

Dunsmuir
•

CRAGS

Valley

WILDERNESS

Road

Lake McCloud

To Redding & Sacramento

LEGEND

Campground ▲	Trail ..._.~..~..			

Road Classification (road network shows only direct route to traiheads)

Interstate ▬▬	State Hwy. ▬▬	Secondary ▬▬	Dirt ═══

CONTENTS

TRIPS BY TYPE & AREA

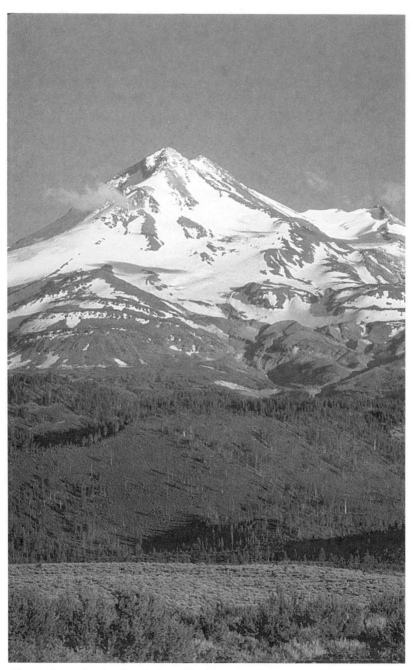

Shasta from the north—Bolam Glacier

INTRODUCTION

RISING OVER 10,000 FEET above its surroundings, Mt. Shasta appears from a distance almost as an apparition, seemingly too huge to be real. The mountain's overwhelming presence makes Joaquin Miller's surreal description, "lonely as God and white as a winter moon," ring as aptly today as it did a century ago. But Mt. Shasta is a very real eminence, not only inspiring the artist and the mystic in us, but offering some of California's most diverse mountain recreation.

From quiet forests and humming glades, to creaking glaciers and windswept parapets, Shasta's slopes set a magnificent stage for excursions ranging from casual rambles to committing challenges. On many given days one can choose between discovering wildflowers along a forest trail, taking ice ax and crampons up to the towering summit, clamping on skis to glide over meadows or swish down a high basin, or jumping on a mountain bike to ride over miles of mountain roads.

The core of this book is a practical guide to this wide range of activities. Although, of course, we encourage anyone with an interest to try any and all of them, each excursion requires its own level of expertise, and readers must judge for themselves what they are ready for, and also judge what the conditions and the weather will allow. At one end of the spectrum, the easier hikes require little more than comfortable footwear and common sense. At the other end, the climbing and ski-mountaineering routes require stamina, technical skill and equipment, and a great sensitivity to the mountain's condition and to oneself. For climbers and skiers without experience on a high mountain like Shasta, this book is no substitute for getting instruction and experience on lesser mountains, where endurance, skill and judgment are less critical. In addition to describing the hikes, climbing routes and ski

1

terrain on Shasta, we've described a number of hikes in the surrounding area, and we've suggested some mountain bike rides as well. In addition, we offer information on white water rafting and kayaking.

In this book we also introduce Mt. Shasta's geology, flora and fauna. This is because, to us, enjoying activities is only half of going to the mountains; the other, more reflective half is coming to know the patterns and processes of the mountain environment. Ideally, during activities and adventures we learn about the environment, and, conversely, while seeking to understand the environment we find adventure and exercise. The two approaches can feed on and balance each other and build more complete experiences and understanding.

DISCOVERY

Mt. Shasta stands in solitary dominance as the most striking mountain in northern California. Its volume—estimated by various geologists at between 80 and 120 cubic miles—makes it, arguably, the largest volcanic peak in the continental United States, and its base-to-summit rise of over 11,000 feet is among the world's largest. Indeed, Mt. Shasta's secondary cone, Shastina, is the third highest summit in the Cascade range. Yet, Mt. Shasta was the last major mountain of the Pacific Northwest to be discovered by European-American explorers. Rainier, Hood, St. Helens, and Baker were all named and mapped before 1800. Shasta, midway between the British settlements at Fort Vancouver at the mouth of the Columbia River, and the Spanish enclaves in San Francisco and Monterey, was not seen by explorers until they had journeyed overland nearly 300 miles from these settlements into unknown territory.

During the summer of 1786 French explorer Jean de la Perouse, completing an exploration of the Pacific, sailed along the northern California coast bound for the Spanish settlements at Monterey. The ship log for September 5 and 6 contained the following entry: "We then perceived a volcano on the summit of the mountain which bore east from us. The flame was very vivid, but a thick fog soon concealed it from our sight. . . ." Historians still disagree over what la Perouse saw. Neither Mt. Shasta nor Lassen Peak can be seen from the Pacific Ocean, but smoke and fire from a major eruption likely could have been visible. la Perouse's maps and journals were sent to Paris before he again set sail, but he was never able to explain in greater detail the volcano he saw, for the famous navigator, his ships, and the crews all disappeared in the south Pacific in 1788.

The early Spaniards in California occasionally sent out expeditions to search for mission sites or to assess the probability of foreign invasion. Two of the first inland explorations were led by Don Luis Arguello. In 1817 and 1821 he sailed up the Sacramento River in small boats, noting the presence of a "very high hill called Jesus Maria," and two mountains he called Los Quates—"the twins." Historians agree that two possibilities exist in terms of this reference: the party may have seen Mt. Shasta and Lassen Peak. The second, more likely, explanation is that they saw Lassen Peak and its adjacent peak, Brokeoff Mountain. Arguello's journals were sparse as to clues about how far north they had travelled, and historians still cannot say with any assurance that these early explorers saw Mt. Shasta.

Hudson Bay Company trapper Peter Skene Ogden left Fort Vancouver on September 12, 1826, journeyed east, then down through central Oregon to encamp at the rich trapping grounds of Klamath Marsh, east of Crater Lake, on December 12. Then, on February 14, 1827, while traveling northwest near the present California-Oregon border, Ogden made his now-famous journal entry: "I have named this river Sastise River. There is a mountain equal in height to Mount Hood or Vancouver, I have named Mt. Sastise. I have given these names from the tribes of Indians."

With this pronouncement, Ogden found favor with historians and was recognized as the discoverer and namer of Mt. Shasta. However, later historians found some interesting discrepancies. Early Hudson Bay Company maps showed

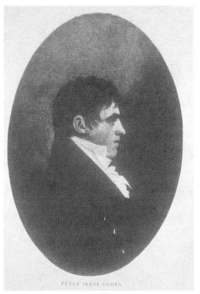

Peter Skene Ogden, credited with the discovery of Mt. Shasta

3

today's Mt. McLoughlin and Rogue River as Mt. Shasta and the Shasta River. "Shasta," a Native American tribe near the mountain, had not been the name of the tribe members for themselves, but the name the Klamath tribe used in referring to them. Later maps portrayed today's Mt. Shasta variously as Mt. Pitt, Mt. Jackson, and Mt. Simpson (as named by Jedediah Smith for George Simpson, governor of the northwest Hudson Bay territory). The 1846 The Oregon Territory wrote: "Pitt Mountain, or, as it is called by the Americans, Mount Jackson, or as by the trappers, Mount Shaste, is said to be 20,000 feet above the level of the sea."

In the early 1980s, archaeologist and historian Jeff Lelande retraced Ogden's route using the original journal records and concluded that Ogden had clearly followed Oregon's Rogue River and had viewed Mt. McLoughlin, naming it "Mt. Sastise." Although Ogden's maps have never been found, history has effectively granted him the title of first European-American discoverer of Mt. Shasta. Whether he actually did remains a mystery to this day.

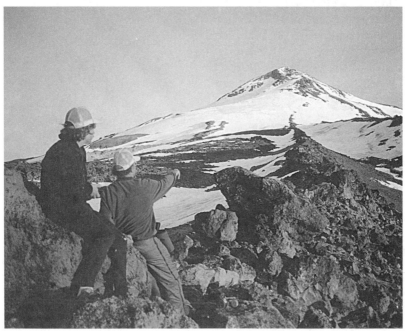

Co-author Michael Zanger pointing out the Hotlum-Bolam Ridge

4

THE MYSTERY

However we mountain lovers try to define our interest, though, most of us find that there's more to Mt. Shasta than we can explain. Something pervasive but not quite tangible draws people to this giant of a mountain. If you approach those who return to Shasta innumerable times—the geologists and botanists, the climbers and skiers—and ask what they like about Shasta besides their pastimes, you'll probably get a rambling affirmation that the mountain is "beautiful" or "impressive, " and that they just like to spend their time on it. While we can't hope to guide readers into ineffable states of mind, we can hint that for many people Mt. Shasta embodies an inspiring and magical presence, yet a presence experienced differently by each person.

Finally, we feel that our responsibility is not only to guide hikers and climbers through their excursions, but to encourage them to leave as little trace of their passing as possible. As a rock-and-ice edifice, Mt. Shasta may be invulnerable, but the mountain's thin, dry soils and high, sterile campsites can be trashed easily by even just one careless visitor. When the goal of minimum impact is honored, simple common sense gives rise to the proper careful practices. Perhaps the most important thing this book can do is to stimulate a more sensitive appreciation for the wonder that is Mt. Shasta. Then Shasta—a bold, attention-getting statement from the natural world—can help us all develop a greater appreciation of and care for the natural world in general.

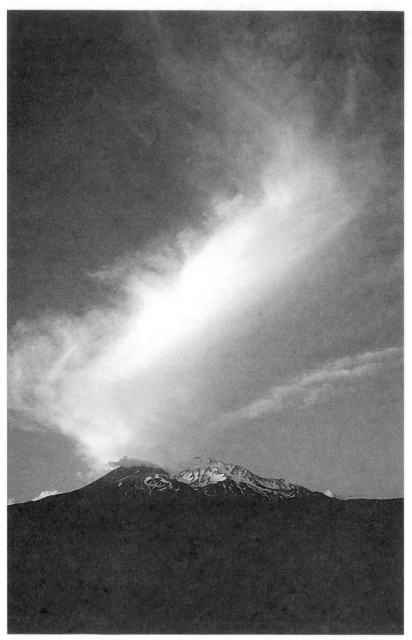

Approaching storm

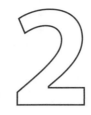

WEATHER

MT. SHASTA is known world-wide for its towering lenticular clouds—those lens-shaped giants that park over the summit like a galactic stack of pancakes. Shasta's winds are also legendary, and during prolonged winter storms aircraft give the mountain a wide berth while climbers and skiers stay indoors. In the summer, billowing cumulus thunderheads can form quickly during afternoons, sometimes producing thunderstorms before sundown.

Nearly all of us who have hiked, camped or climbed have heard the expression, "Mountains make their own weather." In a sense, this is true. But in reality, mountains—and Mt. Shasta is a prime example—are simply showing weather changes *earlier* than the surrounding lowlands.

Certain weather signs on Mt. Shasta give us clues to approaching weather changes and storms. Storms usually move into the Shasta area from the southwest. The first indication of an approaching storm is a change in the wind direction from the prevailing north or east wind to a southwest wind. Wind speed is also likely to increase. Another sign of an approaching storm is the moisture content of the air as indicated by the formation of clouds. The leading edge of a storm usually shows high clouds—cirrus and cirro–stratus. These high clouds thicken and lower as the storm nears. Low level moisture is indicated by Mt. Shasta's famous lenticulars, and other less defined cap clouds. Before storm clouds completely blanket the sky, the top of Mt. Shasta will usually be swathed in a thick cap cloud, which will descend as the storm approaches. Temperatures may be relatively warm before the cap cloud forms, but will fall dramatically once it is in place.

Many hours—or only a few—may elapse from the time a storm's leading edge reaches Shasta until low clouds collect and precipitation begins. If towering cumulus clouds are visible as the storm approaches, the time will usually be short, and thunderstorms may occur with gusty winds, lightning, hail and other associated severe weather.

If you're climbing or hiking on Mt. Shasta below a cap cloud, observing the cloud's actions can be very helpful in forecasting weather changes: If the cap stays above 12,000 feet, the storm may not get worse. Winds will remain high, but the cap cloud may even begin to diminish. If the cap cloud thickens and descends, the storm will probably worsen, and descent from the mountain is advisable. When a storm forms quickly, such as an afternoon thunderstorm, its duration is usually brief—sometimes only a few hours. But if a storm takes one or more days to develop, it can often last for several days before dissipating.

The latest weather information for the Shasta area is available from the following sources:

National Weather Service 24-hour recorded message: (530) 221-5613

The Fifth Season outdoor shop 24-hour climbing report: (530) 926-5555

Mt. Shasta Weather Websites:

www.wunderground.com (click on: Mt. Shasta, CA)

www.weather.com (click on: Mt. Shasta, CA)

www.shastaavalanche.org (many useful links)

www.avalanche.org (click on: Mt. Shasta, CA)

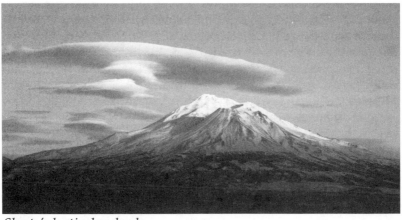

Shasta's lenticular clouds

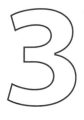

HIKING

HIKING ON SHASTA

MT. SHASTA has a reputation of not offering much to the hiker, but actually there's a lot to choose from. This reputation arose largely because there are fewer than 10 miles of constructed trails on the mountain. But in addition to these trails, hikers' boots have beaten a number of quite evident "trails of use" (aka "scramble trails") to popular destinations, and some abandoned, partly overgrown jeep roads offer scenic, isolated hiking. For those who want to leave the trail, Shasta's open vegetation allows pleasant cross-country hiking and fairly easy route finding, so in this book we suggest a few off-trail excursions.

The mountains near Mt. Shasta offer some excellent hiking also, many with grand panoramas of the Mountain. In the latter part of this chapter we describe some of the better known of these hikes, all of which can be done from a base at Mount Shasta City.

In nearly all the hikes described on Shasta here, you retrace your steps back to the trailhead. The mileages given include the return to the trailhead.

The Forest Service requires a permit for day trips and overnight stays in Mt. Shasta Wilderness. Get one at the Ranger District office in Mt. Shasta (204 W. Alma St., Mt. Shasta, CA 96067; phone (530) 926-4511; hours 8:30-4:00 Mon.-Sat. Outside those hours you can find self-issue permits outside the office). Dogs are not allowed in the Wilderness Area or on Sierra Club Foundation property at Horse Camp.

As of the summer of 2005, the Forest Service had no quota to limit hiking and climbing on Mt. Shasta, although occasional discussions to limit hiker numbers could lead to quotas in the coming years. The agency has, however, included Mt. Shasta in its Recreation Fee Demonstration program. This program, now permanent, has been renamed the Federal Recreation Enhancement Program, and is designed to test the idea of recreational users helping to pay for local maintenance and administration.

As of 2005, a $15 "summit pass" was required for going above an altitude of 10,000 feet on Shasta. Alternatively, the agency offers a $25 pass good for one calendar year. These passes are available at the Forest Service office. The daily passes are also available at self-issue stations at the trailheads. Citizens and permanent residents of the U.S. age 62 or older and possessing the Golden Age Passport, are eligible for a 50% discount on federal recreation use fees for most facilities and services.

The fees collected go toward the general recreation operations of Shasta-Trinity National Forest, including the salaries of the climbing rangers, who do an excellent job of educating climbers and cleaning up after thoughtless individuals. However, it remains to be seen whether this controversial program will treat wilderness recreation the same as other "uses" of the national forests, and whether it will principally pay for the collection of the fees.

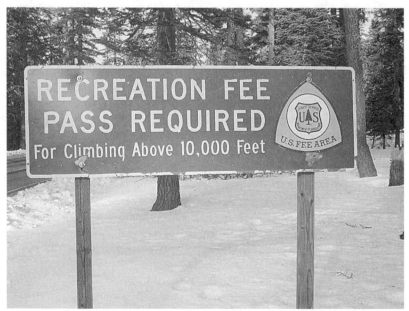

A "summit pass" is now required on Mt. Shasta.

As land managers on Mt. Shasta, both the Forest Service and the Sierra Club Foundation are committed to the belief that wilderness mountains are a precious resource that need the respect and care of all visitors. Both institutions have enlisted the Leave No Trace guidelines as established by the Leave No Trace Center for Outdoor Ethics. This national program seeks to instill a value that wilderness visitors should leave the mountains as unblemished—or better—than when they came. For more information on this program, visit www.lnt.org. Because Mt. Shasta is a popular and rarefied high-altitude environment, as of 2005 the Forest Service requires that all visitors to the Mt. Shasta Wilderness pack out their human waste. Pack-out bags usually are available at the trailheads.

TRAILHEADS

In many of the trailhead driving descriptions, a mileage in **boldface** type gives the distance from the previous mileage. Thus the boldface mileages are a noncumulative log. For example, ". . . after **1.2** miles turn left (W) and drive up a couple . . . after **1.7** miles turn . . ." means that the second turn is 1.7 miles after the first. Mileages in normal type provide additional information.

Much of the access to Mt. Shasta is from Everitt Memorial Highway, which leads from Mount Shasta City up to timberline on the south flank of the mountain. To get to the highway from North Mt. Shasta Blvd., turn northeast onto Alma St. and continue for 0.3 mile, past a right turn and stop sign, to the start of the highway at Mt. Shasta High School.

Getting to trailheads on the north and east sides of Mt. Shasta involves negotiating a network of logging roads. Forest Service maintenance of the routes to the Brewer Creek, Clear Creek and North Gate trailheads is generally adequate for standard passenger vehicles. Signage of the routes to those trailheads is usually adequate but not as reliable. Getting to the other trailheads can involve rougher driving and adventures in routefinding. The trailhead descriptions in this book cover every junction as of spring 2005. Although logging activity has declined in recent years, new logging roads occasionally change the road network on the north and east sides of the mountain.

11

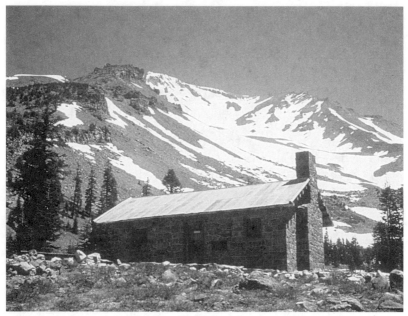

The Sierra Club Foundation's Shasta Alpine Lodge at Horse Camp

Horse Camp (from Bunny Flat)
3.4 miles round trip, moderate

The best-known trail on Shasta, this path takes you to the timberline cabin owned by the Sierra Club Foundation. Anyone may visit the cabin and use its library. The Foundation does charge a small fee for camping here. With Shasta rising directly above it and a fountain of pure spring water piped to it, Horse Camp lures many hikers to stay overnight at one of the established camp spots there.

TRAILHEAD

There are two trails to Horse Camp off Everitt Highway, from Bunny Flat and from Sand Flat. More people take the trail from Bunny Flat, although it is about 0.1 mile longer, because it climbs more gradually, starting 100 feet higher. From Mount Shasta City, Bunny Flat is 10.9 miles up Everitt Highway, and the trailhead is right on the road. There are a large parking area and an outhouse here, as well as stations for wilderness permits, summit passes, and human waste pack-out bags.

DESCRIPTION

With a full view of Mt. Shasta, you start north along the west edge of an expansive dry meadow. Then promptly turn west over a low ridge and hike northwest through other open areas of Bloomer's goldenbush, on the fringes of Shasta red-fir forest. The wide trail (an old road for the first 0.75 mile) jogs north, then continues climbing gently to a broad, open ravine where young red firs lie strewn about. These trees were victims of the large snow avalanches that roar down Avalanché Gulch during heavy winters.

From this ravine the trail turns northwest up the side of a wooded ridge, to reach the trail coming up from Sand Flat. This latter trail has pretty much followed this ridge from the forested trailhead, climbing through a manzanita clearing with logging stumps and then through forest again to this junction.

Now you hike on a steady grade northeast along the flank of the ridge, pausing perhaps to hear the twitters and calls of mountain chickadees and Steller's jays. At the end of the climb a jog northwest heralds your arrival at the meadows of Horse Camp. Here the Sierra Club Foundation posts a summer caretaker, who can answer questions about everything from climbing conditions to the cabin's history, from the latest local environmental controversy to where it's best to camp. The Foundation charges a small fee to camp in the Horse Camp area. Camping is allowed inside the cabin only in emergencies.

Horse Camp is so named because it was here that early-day climbers tethered their horses while ascending Shasta. Above Horse Camp the fir forest gives way to open timberline slopes, luring hikers farther. Behind the cabin the Olberman's Causeway starts climbers up the traditional summit climbing route, and this path makes a nice extension for hikers to follow for a way as well.

SIDE TRIPS FROM HORSE CAMP

For those interested in some cross-country hiking, two particularly scenic destinations from here are Hidden Valley and Green Butte.

Hidden Valley is a broad, perched bench in Cascade Gulch that makes an excellent place from which to look south over seemingly all of California. From the Sierra Club Foundation lodge, look almost due north along the left skyline of Shasta and you'll see a small but striking finger of rock. This pinnacle, Point 9487 on the topo map, lies directly above and south of Hidden Valley.

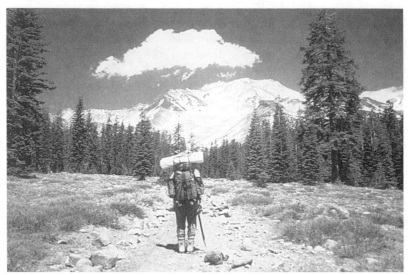

Trail to Horse Camp

From just north of the cabin, you may find the fairly distinct use-trail that now heads toward Hidden Valley. Strike off toward the pinnacle and then climb up sandy, forested slopes to a tiny basin. Continue north, climbing past a few outstanding tall firs and up more sandy slopes, to eventually turn into the drainage of Cascade Gulch. The final stretch to Hidden Valley is an exasperating, traversing climb up a rocky slope to the head of the gulch. But in Hidden Valley you're rewarded with a mostly reliable stream in a *krummholz* "forest." Here Shasta and Shastina loom over you in an amphitheater of high mountain grandeur.

Green Butte is almost due east of Horse Camp, and from its summit you can also look far to the south, with rugged Sargents Ridge towering behind you.

From Horse Camp hike east across the sandy, open drainage of Avalanche Gulch and then start climbing steadily, aiming for the broad, relatively gentle slope in the major ridge to the east. This slope, called an erosion surface, was smoothed by gradual erosion; it has escaped the action of glaciers that have flowed on either side. From this broad slope, hike northeast to near the summit of Point 9365, then turn southeast to descend along the very narrow rock ridge to the summit of Green Butte, so named for its distinctively green rock. Many of the summit rocks are *fulgurites*, rocks fused into glassiness by lightning strikes.

Gray Butte

2.8 miles round trip, easy

This hike takes you through meadow and forest to the panoramic crest of one of Shasta's satellite buttes.

TRAILHEAD

Drive up Everitt Highway 11.4 miles, going past Bunny Flat, and turn into the Panther Meadow campground. Keep left at a couple of campground spurs and park at the east edge of the campground, just below the highway.

DESCRIPTION

Your trail starts east across Panther Meadow, a rich, verdant glade unusual on Mt. Shasta. Particularly strong springs above the meadow keep the ground here saturated, preventing tree growth but providing a rich substrate for subalpine herbs. Different degrees of saturation here favor different plants: the wettest areas adjacent to stream channels are dense with rushes, monkey flowers and swamp onions; most of the meadow is seasonally saturated and dominated by heather, bilberry and laurel; the meadow's drier periphery supports goldenbush and Shasta arnica, although one can see that young mountain hemlocks and Shasta red firs are starting to claim the drier ground. This meadow vegetation is fragile, so please stay on the trail as you cross.

Across the meadow you duck into Shasta red-fir forest and gradually climb on a rocky, dusty track. Continue east along the south base of an unnamed butte, winding your way up to a saddle where a few whitebark pines mix with the firs. Here, 0.6 mile from Panther Meadow campground, an unsigned trail heads northeast for upper South Gate Meadows, while yours leads south and starts a steadily climbing traverse along the east slope of Gray Butte.

As you climb the steady grade, views open up to Red Butte and the flanks of Mt. Shasta. Before long you turn west around the east ridge of Gray Butte, stepping from a thicket of young mountain hemlocks into a mature forest of husky adult trees, perhaps the finest mature hemlock stand in the Shasta area.

Continue climbing steadily under the hemlocks, passing pine-mat manzanita and violets as you arc around the southeast slopes of Gray Butte and gradually approach a dirt road that serves radio facilities atop the butte. You arrive at the open crest of the butte with a panorama across Strawberry Valley to Mt. Eddy and the rest of the Siskiyous and the Trinity Alps. More to the south you see Castle Crags, and beyond the McCloud River country rises Lassen Peak. For full views of Mt. Shasta, you might want to hike northeast up the ridge to Gray Butte's highest point. This has been a famous overlook for the region ever since pioneer photographer Carleton Watkins set up his tripod here in 1870.

Squaw Valley/South Gate Name Changes

Many locations around North America have been named "Squaw," but the word is a vulgarity originating with the Narragansett language. The powers that decide on geographic names are gradually agreeing to remove the word, and, as a place that is sacred to Native American traditions, the slopes of Mt. Shasta are a good place to show respect in this way. In 2005, the Forest Service decided to rename "The Gate" "South Gate," and then rename the parts of "Squaw Valley" on Mt. Shasta "South Gate Meadows." Their signs and their new 2006 maps will show the change immediately, but the topographic maps from the USGS and Wilderness Press will have to wait for new printings to be updated. As of this writing, it is unclear when lower Squaw Valley (hike on page 33) will have a new name.

South Gate Meadows/Squaw Valley
4.4 miles round trip, moderate

Lush green meadows framed by groves of delicate mountain hemlock make Squaw Valley—Shasta's only extensive verdant drainage—one of the mountain's most popular destinations. In respect to Native American terminology, the area has recently been renamed South Gate Meadows, as described above. Although the Forest Service has never constructed a trail here, except for a couple of short sections the track is quite evident. Many people enjoy meeting up with this *de facto* trail after a cross-country loop around Red Butte.

TRAILHEAD

Your trail branches off the previously described Gray Butte Trail, which starts at Panther Meadow. If you like, however, you can shorten the hike by starting from the old Ski Bowl parking lot at the end of Everitt Highway, then hiking cross-country over the saddle north of Point 8332 to meet the trail in the open flats south of South Gate, a rocky defile.

DESCRIPTION

From Panther Meadow take the Gray Butte Trail east for 0.6 mile to a saddle north of Gray Butte. Here the Gray Butte Trail turns south, while your path contours northeast for a short distance. Soon afterward you will rise over a steep, rocky ridgelet, then climb a bit more along the east base of that ridgelet. Next, follow the path on a narrow way through shrubby mountain hemlocks, curving northeast to some slabs that look east to nearby Red Butte.

From these slabs you will wind northeast, crossing a ravine and heading toward broad, open flats below the west walls of Red Butte. The path disintegrates in the dark, loose ash in these flats, but by keeping on a north-northeast bearing you work toward the head of the shallow drainage. This stark, silent basin supports a few ground-hugging plants like knotweed and buckwheat, and numerous wildflowers nodding white blossoms over the dark sand only add to the surreal aura.

Near the head of the shallow drainage you find the trail again and walk through South Gate. A short, steep drop then leads you into the canyon between Red Butte and Sargents Ridge. Now the trail steadily descends into hemlock country, keeping north above the rocky canyon floor. Before long the track turns northeast through a hemlock grove to a stream. You cross another fork or two of the stream and then climb a short way to arrive at upper South Gate Meadows.

Here sedges, heather and various wildflowers grow in a rich carpet beside a perennial brook, fed by a spring that issues from the snowy ramparts of Shasta above. Unlike most drainages on Shasta, the substrate underlying South Gate Creek somehow keeps a steady flow of water flowing on the surface, and "stringer" meadows like this one lie beside the creek well into the forest belt. These meadows—so precious on Shasta—are easily trampled into mud, so please refrain from hiking on them. Some of Shasta's religious groups particularly enjoy these meadows, but unfortunately

17

they often leave stones arranged in public testimony to their religious experience.

Red Butte Loop Variation
(Cross Country)

The trail to South Gate Meadows runs around the north-side of Red Butte. In order to form a loop, many hikers enjoy going around the south side of the butte, returning on the north-side trail.

From the saddle on the Gray Butte Trail (0.6 mile from Panther Meadow), where the trail to South Gate Meadows forks northeast, you'll want to eye the basin to the southeast and plot your course, which will cross the basin below you and climb back up to a prominent bench on the south side of Red Butte. With that bench in mind, strike off east, heading down into fir and hemlock forest and reaching a creek before long at the bottom of the basin.

You'll probably want to head down the basin a short way before starting a steady climb east toward the bench. Stay fairly close to the southern abutments of Red Butte, however, where relatively moderate slopes readily allow you to climb due east. When you arrive at the bench, you break into an expansive, sparsely vegetated meadow, a secluded world of its own. At the meadow's southeast edge a small lake of pooled snow melt remains into early summer.

Hike northeast across the bench, back into a forest edge, and come to a precipitous drop. Without getting too close, veer northwest along the top of the cliff and past its far end, and you'll see a worn path traversing down into a ravine. Follow this path as it crosses the gravelly slope of a small cinder cone, and climb out the other side of the ravine to then contour north. Descending slightly as you traverse north, you'll eventually come to a meadow where a feeder of South Gate Creek keeps the ground soggy year-round.

Here you turn northwest to climb along the southern edge of the meadow, keeping near the talus at the northeast base of Red Butte. Your climb steepens as you re-enter forest and pass the spring that wets the meadow. After a steady climb you reach the rocky canyon between Red Butte and Sargents Ridge, and you can pick up the trail to upper South Gate Meadows. By following it west through South Gate, you can return to the Gray Butte Trail and Panther Meadow.

Clear Creek

4.9 miles round trip, moderate

Although the drive to the trailhead is complex, only a short hike on this trail takes you to spectacular vistas along the rim of Mud Creek Canyon, then on to timberline panoramas of Shasta and its four eastern glaciers.

TRAILHEAD

From McCloud, take Hwy. 89 east **3.0** miles and turn left (N) on paved Pilgrim Creek Road, signed for Mt. Shasta Wilderness Trailheads. Follow this road as it curves northeast, and after **5.3** miles turn left (NW) onto Road 41N15. Go northwest (left) on this road **4.9** miles, to where it intersects Road 31. Continue straight across Road 31, keep left at **0.1** mile, and after **0.5** mile more bear left on 41N25Y. Take this road **1.6** miles through a heavily logged area and veer left. Just **0.2** mile farther turn right, staying on 41N25Y for another **0.6** mile to the trailhead. Along the 3.0 miles from Road 31 there should be Forest Service signs pointing the way to Clear Creek Trailhead.

DESCRIPTION

The Clear Creek Trail evolved from an old jeep road pushed through by four-wheel-drive enthusiasts and woodcutters. Since the designation of the Mt. Shasta Wilderness, the Forest Service has blocked the jeep track and constructed a well-graded hiking path.

The hike starts in a smooth furrow and rises gradually under venerable red firs hung with lime-colored staghorn lichen. A few lazy switchbacks let you enjoy this sylvan enclosure for not quite a mile, then deliver you to the east rim of Mud Creek Canyon at about 6900 feet. Here the forest opens to views of Shasta's skyline, with Shastarama Point and Thumb Rock above the Konwakiton Glacier. On Shasta's eastern flank hang the Watkins and Wintun glaciers, and in the depths of its canyon, Mud Creek plummets over two powerful waterfalls.

Mud Creek Canyon is Shasta's largest and oldest canyon, dating from the proto–Mt. Shasta of a few hundred thousand years ago. During snowy epochs glaciers have filled the canyon, transporting debris and helping to excavate its grand depths. During warm spells in the 1920's and '30's, the Mud Creek Glacier steadily disintegrated, and issued outburst floods. These spilled out of the canyon and into the town of McCloud, and it is said that silty outwash from the largest ones clouded San Francisco Bay.

Staying near the canyon edge, you climb gradually on a roller-coaster course. As you reach the area above the confluence of Clear Creek and Mud Creek far below, you leave most of the firs behind and enter whitebark-pine country, where Clark nutcrackers squawk at your intrusion into their domain. You can follow the track into the *krummholz* zone, to near 8300 feet. At this height Clear Creek's drainage broadens and allows one to traverse west a quarter mile to a surprisingly verdant destination, the source springs of Clear Creek.

Brewer Creek
4.0 miles round trip, moderate

Constructed in 1986, this trail offers well-graded access to timber-line on Shasta's less-visited east slopes. Although the drive to the trailhead is dusty and fairly complex, at this writing the roads are passable to any car and are well signed. The hike rewards one with pleasant walking through unusual forests of whitebark pines, good views of Shasta and its glaciers, and access to summer ski slopes and glacier climbing.

TRAILHEAD

Allow 1½ hours from the Mount Shasta City. As for the Clear Creek Trailhead, take Hwy. 89 east from McCloud for **3.0** miles and turn left onto Pilgrim Creek Road. After **7.4** miles on this paved road turn left onto Road 19, which should be signed for Brewer Creek, North Gate and Military Pass. Continue on 19, bear left at **2.9** miles, right at **1.5** miles more, and at **2.6** miles farther come to 42N02. Turn left here and climb a steeper, bumpier road, keeping left at **0.9** mile and again at **0.8** mile farther. This second left puts you on 42N10, and on this you keep right at **0.3** mile, and contin-ue uphill through switchbacks for **1.9** miles more to the road end, 22.7 miles from Hwy. 89, at 7250 feet.

DESCRIPTION

You start hiking south, climbing gently up a track barely dis-cernible as an old roadbed. Where the old road switchbacks, the trail continues south, and then it turns west to regain the roadbed and turns south again. Half a mile from the trailhead the road ends for good, and you start a series of long, lazy switchbacks that take you from an open red-fir forest into a parkland of whitebark pines. Hardy wildflowers dot the ashy soil between whitebarks, including violets, phlox and Shasta knotweed.

After several switchbacks your trail takes a fairly steady course south, still gradually climbing through extensive stands of burly whitebarks. Now, however, you get full views of Shasta, including the Wintun and Hotlum glaciers. The track crosses a few dry ravines, then comes to the fairly reliable flows of Brewer Creek. Snow will provide a bridge across this creek until at least early July, although take care that such a bridge is thick enough.

From Brewer Creek the trail contours south **0.5** mile to meet an old jeep road. Built illegally by 4-wheel-drive enthusiasts, this road is traceable west to 8300 feet, and beyond where it fades out, skiers and snowboarders can find summer snow to *schuss* on, typically into August. If you follow the road downhill (E) **0.1** mile you come to a fork. The southbound branch curves to the top of a small sandy ridge, and from there heads uphill southwest and west, continuing for another **1.5** sandy miles to over 9000 feet, petering out among the highest, most dwarfed *krummholz* whitebarks.

Ash Creek Falls (Cross-Country)

From the Brewer Creek Trail an experienced hiker can trek to Ash Creek Falls, Shasta's prettiest waterfall. The 2.5-mile round trip from the Brewer Creek Trail requires some cross-country route finding and scrambling.

From the old jeep road atop the sandy ridge mentioned above, contour south and drop into a large, dry ravine. Climb back out of the ravine and contour around the next ridge at the 7800-foot level. Curve west at that contour, and you'll soon pass beside a drop from where the falls are partly visible. The best views are to be had from across the canyon, however, and to reach them you'll have to angle down to cross the stream above the falls. Take extreme care to find the easiest way down this slope; if you are on route, only a very short cliff near the bottom will require some scrambling. Through late summer, deep snow forms a sturdy, convenient bridge over the creek, and once across you can reach viewpoints by climbing directly upslope through a band of whitebarks.

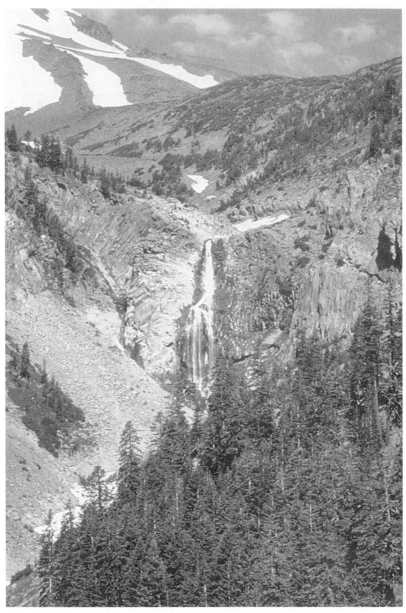

Ash Creek Falls

North Gate
6.5 miles round trip, difficult

In the 1980s this trail was just a boot track worn in by climbers heading to the Hotlum and Bolam glacier routes. With extra traffic and some construction from the Forest Service, now it's a defined trail and a great choice for either a dayhike or an overnight to the panoramic knolls and moraines below the glaciers.

TRAILHEAD

Access roads are somewhat complex and rough; allow at least an hour. From Mount Shasta City, drive north on I-5 to central Weed. At Weed's only stoplight take Hwy. 97 north and after **12.8** miles turn right (SE) onto the Military Pass Road. A historical marker here commemorates this road as a pioneer settler's wagon train route. Continue on this primary dirt road, crossing under railroad tracks, and **4.8** miles from the highway keep left. Continue through curves that trend generally south-southeast for another **3.5** miles to where you turn right onto road 42N17. After another **0.1** mile, keep to your left, and continue climbing for a bumpy **0.6** mile more to the trailhead located in an old clearcut at 6920 feet.

DESCRIPTION

The trail begins by climbing a gully southwest through the clearcut, then enters prime Shasta red-fir forest. Before long, the path steepens up a ravine in the shade of the stately trees, but soon the angle eases as it enters the realm of whitebark pines. Here some of the most magnificent whitebarks you'll find anywhere grow—stout, proud trees that nevertheless show the golden wood where the elements killed the growing tissue. As you travel higher, on your right you will see a swath of these whitebarks laid flat by an avalanche that roared off the steep slope to the south in the heavy winter of 1997.

The sandy track continues climbing gradually through a defile between the avalanche slope and Point 8852, which is a small, recently formed dacite dome. You soon leave the trees behind as you curve south and climb a steady, steep grade into a broader, rockier valley, while the view of Mt. Shasta's most symmetrical facet comes closer with every step. Soon you'll hear and then see a reliable stream tumbling through the rocks.

At about 9500 feet you'll cross the west side of the stream, and then you'll start to see bivouac and tent sites cleared on the little benches in this area. From this height, distant views to the northwest open up over the debris-mounds of Shasta Valley to Preston Peak and the Siskiyous, and to the north over much of the southern Oregon, including Mt. McGloughlin and Klamath Falls.

If you continue climbing, the track will take you to snowline, at about 10,000 feet. An ice ax and stout boots are recommended for ventures onto the snowfields. Whether you camp or turn back for the trailhead, please take extra care to preserve the purity of the snow-melt stream here.

Whitney Falls
3.4 miles round trip, moderate

This casual hike takes you to a good viewpoint **0.3** mile from Whitney Falls, a free fall of about 250 feet. Although most of the hike follows an abandoned jeep trail, open scenery and solitude make it a pleasant excursion. During midsummer this sunny trail can be baking hot.

TRAILHEAD

From the Weed stoplight drive north on Hwy. 97 **10.3** miles to unsigned Bolam Road. If you come to paved County Road A12, which branches north, you've gone 0.3 mile too far on Hwy. 97. On fairly good quality Bolam Road, keep driving south, avoiding an eastbound (left) road at **0.2** mile from Hwy. 97 and another **0.8** mile farther. Another **0.5** mile farther, continue straight across railroad tracks and maintain a southbound course past a couple of other forks to reach the end of the road, 3.7 miles from Hwy. 97. In 1997 a rock slide buried the trailhead and the start of the trail in five feet of debris, but it is easy to hike over the debris and get onto the trail.

DESCRIPTION

Begin by crossing Bolam Creek's dry wash just west of the trailhead, and then turn south onto the jeep road on the west side of this shallow drainage. Phlox, sulphur flower and paintbrush dot this sandy track, and scattered Jeffrey pines, antelope brush and mountain mahogany thinly cover the surrounding hills. Half a mile from the trailhead your path switchbacks up out of the drainage into full view of Shasta and the Bolam Glacier, and to the north you see across Shasta Valley to the northern Siskiyous.

You continue south along the west rim of Bolam Creek's dry ravine for a way, then bend east to climb a couple of switchbacks. These take you south back across the drainage to a steady climb to another switchback. At this switchback a worn-in use trail heads off west into a ravine shaded by a grove of Jeffrey pines and white firs. This path will take you to the Whitney Falls overlook.

From the shaded ravine your use trail climbs steeply around a small ridge, then turns south a short distance to the brink of the impressively eroded canyon of Whitney Creek. The falls plunge off an overhanging cliff at the head of the canyon, and if you listen carefully you'll hear rocks, gravel and mud clattering over the falls; Whitney Falls is anything but a clear stream, for glacial silt and Shasta's unstable ashy debris readily dissolve into the flow. During recent hot summers the Whitney Glacier has released outburst floods (see the "Geology" Chapter) that have poured over the falls and continued downstream to damage property beyond Hwy. 97. The loose canyon walls below you show ample evidence of undercutting by these and previous floods.

Circum-Shasta Hike
25-35 miles, difficult

Hiking around Mt. Shasta is arguably the best way to get to know the mountain. In fact, John Muir wrote:

... far better than climbing [Mt. Shasta] is going around its warm fertile base, enjoying its bounties like a bee circling around a bank of flowers.... As you sweep around so grand a centre the mountain itself seems to turn.... One glacier after another comes into view, and the outlines of the mountain are ever changing.

The first Shasta circumnavigation was completed in the summer of 1898 by Dr. C. Hart Merriam and other members of the U.S. Biological Survey. Merriam, a central figure in American natural history, named Diller Canyon for geologist Joseph Diller, and finalized his "life-zone" theory of plant and animal distribution during this trip.

Relatively few people take this ultimate Shasta backpack, partly because it's a fairly committing endeavor, with no trail to follow. In route finding, strenuousness and terrain, it should be considered

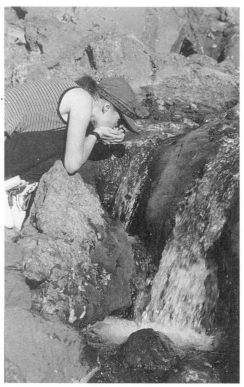

North side of Shasta

a moderate-but-long mountaineering endeavor. Carrying an ice ax and knowing how to self-arrest can be important in the early season high around Shastina. Shasta's relatively open slopes help make route finding fairly easy, but soft, ashy underfooting occasionally gets tedious. One needs to plan the hike carefully to camp at water sources, and to find passages across some of the canyons. However, crossing the toes of several of Shasta glaciers offers superb views, and the short side trips to view various waterfalls, in particular Whitney and Ash Creek falls, are well worth the extra time.

With these cautions in mind, confident backpackers who are comfortable with occasional scrambling should not be deterred from taking one of California's finest backcountry hikes. Very fit hikers can complete the route in four days, and five would be comfortable for most backpackers.

Different hikers choose to circle the mountain at different elevations. A clockwise direction, usually beginning and ending at the Sierra Club Foundation cabin at Horse Camp, is preferred: water sources, campsites, and scenery continually improve in this direction, and most of the tiresome scree is dealt with initially. There are many route variations, especially on the mountain's west flanks, but most hikers stay near the 8000 foot level—approximately treeline. What follows is a *general* description of the possibilities, with mention of key canyon crossings and important campsites.

Starting from Horse Camp, you can stay low, perhaps planning a first camp at Cascade Gulch or Diller Canyon. In dry years these canyons might not offer water, although you can always count on finding snow to melt in Diller Canyon. An alternative route is to go high and spend the first night in Hidden Valley, where water is always available. This enables a higher traverse around Shastina, over spurs 9363 and 9084. Staying high gives you a wonderfully scenic and somewhat shorter route, but it takes you across a couple of trying scree slopes, and you have to negotiate some short cliff bands, 0.25 mile south of Diller Canyon and about 0.75 mile north of it. In any case, be aware that it's a long way around Shastina between good water sources—potentially all the way from Cascade Canyon to Bolam Creek.

To traverse the Graham Creek–Bolam Creek area, it's best to avoid the morainal hills below the Whitney and Bolam glaciers by going somewhat high across the terminus of the Whitney Glacier. There are small grassy areas and springs for camping west of the Whitney Glacier toe, but they can be difficult to find. For those who go high, a reliable camp awaits in the basin below the Bolam Glacier, at about 9600 feet. From this camp it's best to descend along the east side of Bolam Creek to treeline.

In the North Gate vicinity, most hikers contour south of Point 8852, and gradually lose elevation as they continue east. Another option is to climb over the morainal benches near Point 9535, where there's excellent camping on flat, sandy ground, and almost always snowmelt. To continue east off these benches, descend a sandy gully through some cliff bands east-southeast of Point 9535 and contour towards Gravel Creek. Those who are relatively high will find difficulty in crossing Gravel Creek's canyon. The canyon walls consist of steep, unstable ash with boulders perched on it. Members of a party must take special care to avoid knocking rocks onto one another, and not to climb directly below or above one another. Below 7500 feet the canyon walls are safer and not as high.

The next key point is Ash Creek right above the falls. To get there, hike through whitebark parklands near the 8000-foot level across Brewer Creek (reliable and clear). Contour around the ridge just north of the falls at 7800 feet and then cut back west to descend into the canyon above the falls. An 8-foot cliff on this descent requires some scrambling. Solid snow—avalanche debris—usually offers a convenient bridge across Ash Creek until late in summer. On the south side of the canyon, climb directly upslope through a band of whitebarks.

Cold Creek, Pilgrim Creek and Clear Creek are all reliable and silt-free. Contour around Clear Creek's canyon at about 7800 feet to set up for the crucial crossing of intimidating Mud Creek Canyon. From around 7700 feet on the canyon rim, drop straight into the canyon on a loose, sandy rib, at the uppermost grove of full-size firs, just up-canyon from a bare landslide area. Near the canyon bottom, again take special care to avoid sending rocks onto partners. Cross Mud Creek a couple of hundred yards above the falls, and climb directly up a steep, faint drainage to get back out of the canyon. This exit is important; large rocks offer reliable stepping stones to the rim. From the southwest rim of the canyon, a course that contours near 7800 feet will take you around Red Fir Ridge to South Gate Creek. The lush meadows are among the nicest campsites on the mountain. From here you can traverse north of Red Butte on an excellent trail through South Gate to Panther Meadows or the old Ski Bowl. Return to Everitt Highway.

HIKING NEAR SHASTA

The mountains surrounding Mt. Shasta also offer excellent hiking trails. Some feature the great volcano as a backdrop, and all explore terrain beautiful in its own right. Three general areas beckon: the McCloud River country, south and east of McCloud; the Castle Crags, west of Dunsmuir; and the Trinity-Sacramento highlands, south and southwest of Mt. Shasta.

McCloud River Preserve
5.2 miles round trip, easy

Most of the McCloud River drainage has been logged over, and dams have stilled the river's tumbling waters in its lower and upper reaches. But a major stretch of its inner canyon remains a refuge of wilderness, because Bay Area aristocrats bought the land from Central Pacific Railroad for a retreat. In 1973 they donated their upper holdings to The Nature Conservancy, and now much of this corridor has become a wonderful spot for hikers and, especially, fly fishermen (limited to 10 anglers at one time).

TRAILHEAD

From the town of McCloud, turn south off of Hwy. 89 at the service station, onto Squaw Valley Road. Continue on this for **9.2** miles, and then keep right near a boat ramp at McCloud Reservoir. After curving for **2.2** miles above the reservoir, veer right at a sharp turn onto a dirt road signed AH-DI-NA. After **0.6** mile keep left, and after another **1.8** miles keep straight through a junction. Continuing past the spur to Ah-Di-Na Campground, after **4.4** miles stay right. The trailhead is **0.2** mile farther.

DESCRIPTION

The hike starts out across a tributary creek and descends to a forested flat near the river where The Nature Conservancy houses a manager. Please sign in here, and pick up a pamphlet that introduces you to the area's ecology and to Wintu Indian lore via a short interpretive path.

From the manager's flat the trail heads into a botanical wonderland, wandering down-canyon under the shade of Douglas-fir, dogwood, vine and big-leaf maples, and black and canyon oaks.

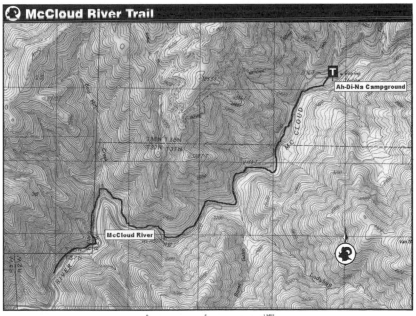

Frequent forest openings with western azalea, deer brush, elder-berry and chokecherry let you marvel at the surrounding canyon, an impressive if small wilderness that supports wolverines, mountain lions, spotted owls, bald eagles and other animals no longer common. Rattlesnakes can also be numerous and active here, so it can be smart to hike with long pants, a walking stick, and a wary ear and eye. Never far away, the river alternately rif-fles and pools, tempting hikers to swim and anglers to wet a line.

The McCloud River is renowned among fly fishermen as one of the hottest spots in California for wily native rainbow and intro-duced brown trout. Until the 1980s it was the southernmost refuge of the Dolly Varden char (also known as bull trout), a generally northern salmonid that survives only in chilly waters. Though the Ice Age ended over 10,000 years ago, the Dolly Varden stayed on in the McCloud because this river derives mostly from cold, pro-fuse springs of Mt. Shasta snowmelt. Unfortunately, the reservoir above the preserve seems to have gradually damaged the char's habitat by warming the water and diverting much of the flow. Also, competing introduced species have expanded upstream from Shasta Lake reservoir. Now the McCloud's Dolly Varden are extinct.

Nearly a mile from the trailhead you come to a fork in the trail, where a shortcut climbs gradually over a knoll to rejoin the river-side trail about a quarter mil0 down. As you tour down-canyon, you pass through occasional rocky openings of greenschist and limestone. Here you especially need to take care to stay clear of poison oak near the trail. Your trail gradually curves with the river, north then south, crossing Bald Mountain Creek on the way. A bit farther it emerges from forest near Boundary Creek and the "Big Bend" in the McCloud. About 0.3 mile beyond you come to trail's end; below here The Nature Conservancy reserves the river and the canyon for nature alone, plus occasional scientific study.

The Nature Conservancy depends on private donations to manage its preserves. If you would like to donate money or to vol-unteer, contact it at:

The McCloud River Preserve
P.O. Box 409785
McCloud, CA 96057
(530) 926-4366

The Nature Conservancy
Market Street, 3rd Floor
San Francisco, CA 94103
(415) 777-0487
www.nature.org

McCloud River Falls

2.9 miles round trip, easy

This easy walk along the McCloud River above Lake McCloud visits prime swimming holes and three elegant waterfalls.

TRAILHEAD

From Mt. Shasta, drive east on Hwy. 89 through the town of McCloud. At 5.7 miles past McCloud, turn right at the paved McCloud River loop road, then keep right to reach the parking lot near the lower falls. The hike starts from a constructed overlook here.

DESCRIPTION

Stairs lead down to a basalt bench, where the river plunges 10 to 15 feet and washes through a very deep pool. The Wintun named this short cataract as the "falls that stop salmon." Swimmers enjoy diving here, and though the water is refreshing on a hot day, most are surprised by the chilly entry. The water temperature stays cool

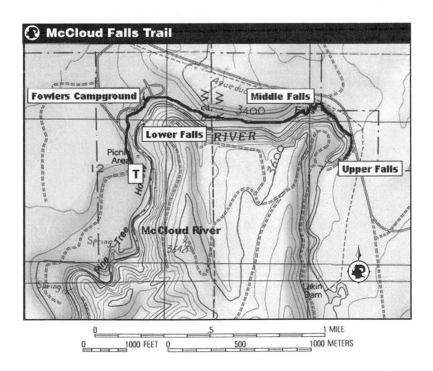

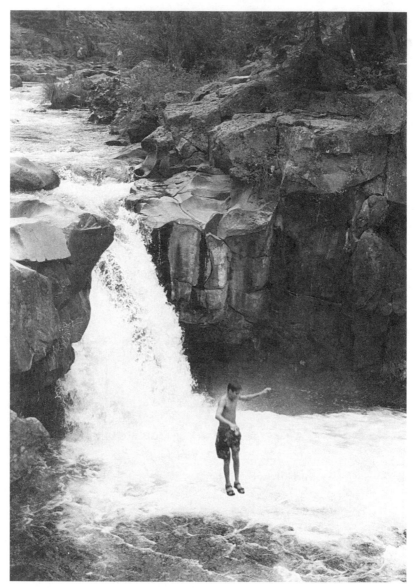

Boy jumping into pool at lower falls

because much of this water starts its journey as Mt. Shasta snow melt and flows underground through porous volcanic bedrock on its way here. From this falls head upstream and catch a paved path that weaves a couple of switchbacks up to a higher bench. Keep right on this path as it curves along the rim of the bench, and walk past the fringe of Fowler's Campground.

At the east end of the campground the pavement ends and the trail takes a quiet, flat course beneath Douglas-firs and alders. Through the woods you can see eroding cut banks across the river, including some hoodoo towers, where perched boulders rest atop spires of sediments protected from erosion by the cap of stone. A growing roar and a driving mist announce your approach to Middle Falls, and soon you reach a switchback where everyone scrambles over slippery talus to get a riverside view. This falls pours off a 35-foot-high cliff in a curtain 80 feet wide.

Back on the trail, take a switchback uphill and follow a couple more hairpins to stairs that gain the top of the cliffs and a splendid overlook of Middle Falls. You also might see ospreys from here. The cliff-edge path continues southeast past manzanita and ponderosa pine, and an easy 0.4 mile of additional walking brings you to Upper Falls. Here the whole river churns through a polished, curvy basalt slot before launching some 60 feet into the pool below. There is no railing here, and anyone tempted to get a full view down the falls risks a quick death. Behind the trees lies a large dirt parking lot. To return to your car, retrace your steps and enjoy the waterfalls again.

Squaw Valley Creek
7.1 miles loop trip, moderate

The lower canyon of Squaw Valley Creek holds one of the finest sanctuaries of old-growth forest in interior northern California, thanks to the concerns of the McCloud River Club aristocrats in the 1950s, and later to the Sierra Club. Walking through this low-elevation refuge makes for a pleasant day any time of year. During summer's heat, many secluded pools await for a cooling swim. Spring or fall will be colorful with, respectively, flowers or autumn brilliance, and on a drizzly winter day under an umbrella these native woods inspire reverence. At this writing a last section of the trail is not yet finished, and so hikers have retraced their steps to the trailhead. But with the long-delayed construction expected to be completed during the summer of 2006, a loop hike will be possible.

TRAILHEAD

From Mt. Shasta, drive east on Hwy. 89 **11** miles to McCloud, and turn right (south) at the service station onto Squaw Valley Road. Take this country drive for **6.2** miles to a right turn onto a prominent dirt road (39N21) signed for Squaw Valley Creek and Cabin Creek/PCT. Follow this for **3.0** miles, and just after crossing a bridge park in the large lot at 2800 feet.

DESCRIPTION

Step down off the parking area and promptly you'll cross a footbridge over Cabin Creek. Ignore a fisherman's path heading up this stream, and turn left to follow the much larger flow of Squaw Valley Creek, waters which originate in Mt. Shasta's snow melt. The first cascade-and-pool sequence is just downstream. Anglers often try their luck here for both rainbows and browns, up to the daily limit of two. Across the canyon a ghost forest stands above brush, the result of a careless smoker in 1990. About a quarter mile down the canyon you meet the Pacific Crest Trail where it spans the creek on a sturdy bridge. Join the PCT for a short distance while contouring downstream, to where the PCT turns uphill to resume its westward course.

As you continue downstream, impressive Douglas-firs, incense cedars and a few ponderosa pines tower above with a shading canopy, and live oaks and black oaks shaggy with moss thrive in an open understory. The path generally descends or contours near the stream, but at one point it ascends some to overlook the curving creek from a limestone outcrop.

An ambling half-mile after this you are back down by the bank, where water-polished basalt juts into the current, offering a nice peninsula to rest on, assuming the spring runoff has diminished. Dogwoods here add white blossoms in spring, and in the fall their leaves compete with vine maples in crimson and yellow. You have to remember, though, to keep an eye toward the ground for occasional shoots of poison oak.

Contour around minor side canyons and spurs, and 1.8 miles from the car you reach a small bench nearly encircled by a broad, quiet arc in the stream. One can camp on this bench, where with some luck one might see or hear a northern spotted owl, the politically important bird that needs mature forests, and whose federal endangered status helped spare this canyon from logging.

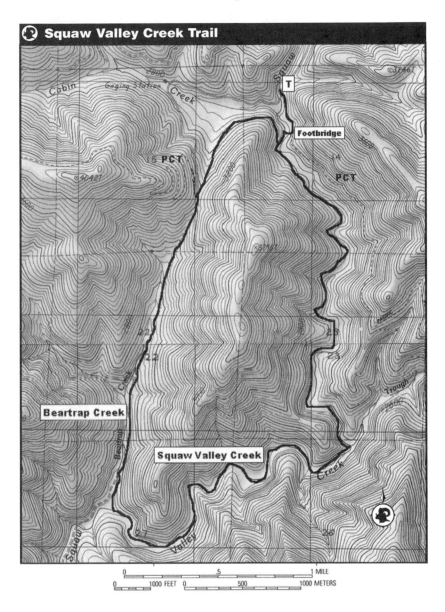

Squaw Valley Creek Trail

From the end of the stream's arc, the path descends gradually, passing old burned trunks reminding that fire has been a periodic visitor here since well before Smokey's time. Barely in view behind oaks and Douglas-firs, the stream quietly collects before pouring over a waterfall and into another pool. From there your path climbs some over a minor spur thick in black oaks, and turns onto warmer south-facing slopes where live oaks dominate. Behind dense cover now, the current tumbles over a second waterfall, while the path works down-canyon on a ledge excavated in metamorphic outcrops. Soon the track reaches outcrops that, in early 2006, are yet to have a trail bed cleared through them.

With trail completion scheduled for later in 2006 by the Forest Service, though, you'll be able to continue down-canyon another 1.3 miles and turn north up Beartrap Creek. Soon after turning up-canyon, you'll meet the McCloud Club's private road, which is closed to public traffic. Hike this road up-canyon for 1.5 miles through more superb forest, and you'll come again to the Pacific Crest Trail. Take the PCT east for 0.7 mile, around a spur and back down to the Squaw Valley Trail, completing a loop 0.2 mile below where you parked your car.

CASTLE CRAGS

Steeped in history and legend, the rugged granite of Castle Crags is a jagged contrast to symmetrical volcanic Mt. Shasta just across Strawberry Valley. During the early 1850s a brief but unsuccessful gold rush strained both the environment and relations with the Indians living near the Crags.

Joaquin Miller, later known as "the poet of the Sierra," lived for a time in the area chronicling the history, and helped to perpetrate legends of lost Indian gold. In 1855 a battle was fought with the Indians in which Miller claimed to have been wounded. It was likely the last time in the West in which Indians relied exclusively upon bows and arrows. Battle Mountain, an impressive 1500-foot wall on the west side of the Crags, was named for this conflict.

For many years pioneers and settlers traveled through the area on the old California-Oregon trail. In 1886 the Southern Pacific Railroad was put through the Sacramento River canyon, effectively opening the country to mining and lumbering. Resorts prospered near the Crags' many mineral springs, and Castle Rock Mineral Water became famous throughout California. Diligent efforts by a far-sighted local citizenry resulted in the acquisition of the Crags in 1933 by the newly formed California State Parks System. In 1984, 7300 acres of National Forest land adjacent to the Park were designated as a federal wilderness area.

Castle Crags State Park has 64 drive-in family campsites and a special walk-in area for backpackers and Pacific Crest Trail hikers.

Picnicking, hiking, fishing and swimming are the most popular activities; you can enjoy several miles of improved trails within the Park, including 2 miles of riverside trail. The Pacific Crest Trail runs through the Park yielding magnificent views of the Crags from varying perspectives, and some outstanding glimpses of nearby Mt. Shasta. The Crags are also a relatively unused venue for rock climbing. You can obtain climbing information at Park Headquarters or at The Fifth Season outdoor shop in Mount Shasta. For further information:

Castle Crags State Park
P.O. Box 80
Castella, CA 96017-0080
(530) 235-2684

Castle Dome
5.6 miles round trip, moderate

The Castle Crags startle most drivers on I-5, as the granite parapets, spires, pinnacles and domes rise above the surrounding hills with a surreal grandeur. The popular hike described here brings one to some spectacular views right among the crags. While the hike is quite an inspiring climb, it's but an introduction to "The

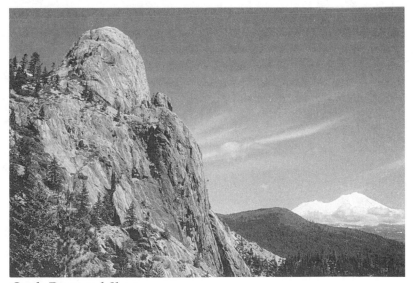

Castle Dome and Shasta

Crags." Acres and acres of towers and hidden valleys extend behind what one can see. Many of the crags are known to climbers, and some of the high valleys were the last hideouts for Indians.

A campground and the first half of the trail are in a state park, while most of Castle Crags is national forest wilderness. At present no permit is needed to enter Castle Crags Wilderness, but there is a fee to enter the State Park.

TRAILHEAD

From I-5 take the Castella exit, which is 14 miles south of Mount Shasta and 47 miles north of Redding. On the west side of the freeway, keep right and drive past the Castella Tavern and post office, and keep right again to reach the entrance to Castle Crags State Park. Here there is a day-use charge, which also admits one to the showers in the campground. From the entrance station follow trailhead signs for Castle Dome through the campground onto a steeply switchbacking road, which ends at a trailhead parking lot 1.3 miles from the entrance station.

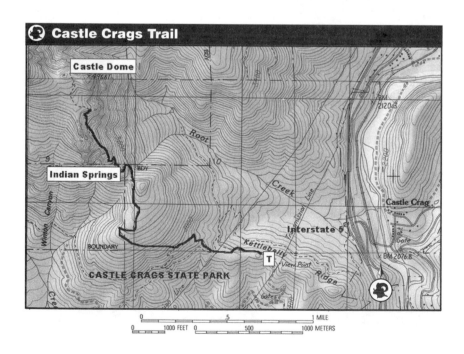

DESCRIPTION

From the road's last curve your hike starts west on a broad, flat path in the shade of Douglas-firs and black oaks. In 0.3 mile you come to a junction from which a spur trail contours north for 0.6 mile to Root Creek. Your trail continues west and starts climbing, soon arriving at a junction with the Pacific Crest Trail at a clearing for power lines atop Kettlebelly Ridge. You continue climbing west, back into the forest.

After a couple of steep switchbacks the path rises gradually, turning north around a ridge and climbing past your first close-up view of the crags. To the southwest another group of cliffs, Grey Rocks, pokes up as well. You next arrive at a forested saddle from where a spur trail contours off west for 0.3 mile to Indian Springs, a refreshing oasis shaded by big-leaf maples.

From this junction the trail continues north to a dramatic vista of the 1200-foot east face of Castle Dome, looming over the Root Creek drainage, and Mt. Shasta beyond. From here you turn back into the woods for another quarter mile before coming upon outlying spires. The trail switchbacks and weaves over a craggy notch, then continues to climb steadily beneath a series of 100-300-foot walls. A long, rising traverse brings you to a few rocky switchbacks and, climbing these brings you to the shoulder below the south face of Castle Dome.

West of this manzanita-covered shoulder some of the other spectacular crags rise in all their bold jaggedness. The Castle Crags are an uplift of granodiorite fairly similar to that of the Sierra, but for reasons unknown lying some distance from that range. Geologists speculate that the Crags—and the entire Klamath region—originally were connected to the present north end of the Sierra, but if so they were long ago displaced to the west by some as yet undiscovered faulting.

The maintained trail ends at this shoulder below Castle Dome. However, a use trail winds farther north-northwest through the manzanita, becoming a deeply eroded rut where one must clamber over exposed roots. This rut brings you to the saddle west of Castle Dome, where you can wander among some outcrops and look over the headwaters of Root Creek, an extensive palace of slabs and spires. Take care in scrambling over any rocks, for in places the potential fall is very serious. A fenced overlook right at the base of Castle Dome offers a particularly breathtaking view.

Castle Lake–Mt. Bradley

10.8 miles round trip, moderate–difficult

Surprisingly uncrowded, this route climbs from a large subalpine lake, past another smaller lake, to a spectacularly scenic ridge walk.

TRAILHEAD

From downtown Mount Shasta drive southwest across I-5 (on the overpass of the main Mount Shasta exit) to a "T" at Old Stage Road. Turn left (SW) and after **0.3** mile veer right, toward Lake Siskiyou. Continue across the dam at Lake Siskiyou, and after just a few hundred yards turn left onto Castle Lake Road. This road climbs **7.1** miles to Castle Lake.

Although swimmers, anglers, and sunbathers flock to Castle Lake on summer weekends, the enclosing granite cliffs and forests still reflect in the lake's clear waters, and the basin still suggests a

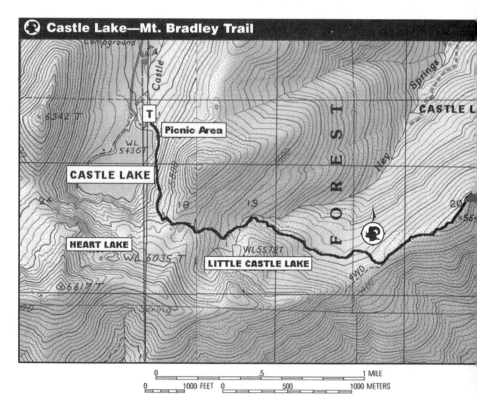

High Sierra-like setting. Scientists have studied the lake intensively, finding among other things that the lake supports many fish partly because a couple of lakeside alder groves add nitrogen to the waters.

DESCRIPTION

From the very end of the parking lot, walk east across the lake's outlet and pick up your signed trail as it leads south near the lake's east shore. The path promptly starts climbing among open groves of Shasta red fir and western white pine here, letting you look down on Castle Lake's shimmering surface. Keep left at an unmarked spur, and continue climbing steeply southeast. Your climb soon takes you out of the trees to rocky going through a bonanza of seasonal wildflowers. Brodiaea, mountain pride, stonecrop and mariposa lilies grow among the rusty metamorphic outcrops where you top out at the crest of Castle Lake's basin.

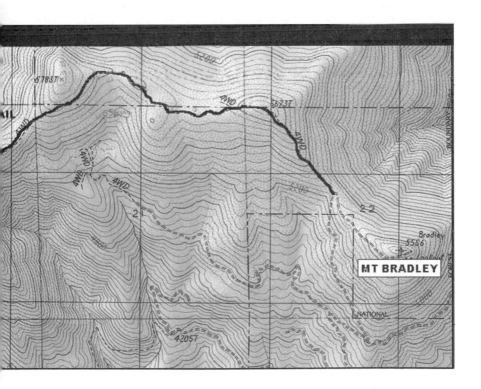

From the saddle here the trail turns east past a small ephemeral pond and starts a steep descent through a dense fir stand. The descent brings you into a verdant meadow, and across this glade under a bluff lies Little Castle Lake. You continue east past the short spur to this lake and hike across the outlet stream. A roller-coaster section of trail then takes you across broken slopes into a fairly level, dense forest. The trail is a bit hard to follow here, but tree blazes mark the way. Tree-watchers might notice among the firs a specimen of "weeping," or Brewer, spruce, a fairly rare tree found only in the Klamath-Trinity region.

In this forest the trail abruptly turns south almost straight upslope, and then emerges onto the ridgetop above with a stunning view of the Castle Crags. Few people venture into the northern crags you see from here, and though the view is extensive it includes only about one-fifth of the Crag's total complex.

On the ridgetop trail, wide to serve as a firebreak, head northeast, and before long the view opens entirely to include Mt. Shasta, Lassen Peak, Mt. Eddy (across Strawberry Valley from Shasta) and Lake Siskiyou. One can continue along the ridgetop, rising and descending in and out of occasional Jeffrey-pine groves, to join a road that continues for 0.6 mile to an old Forest Service lookout at Mt. Bradley, 3.4 miles from where you first gained the ridge.

When hiking back along the ridgetop, keep alert for the trail which descends northwest off the ridge back into the woods because an extension of the ridgeline path continues southwest and disappears into the brush at the head of the drainage to the south.

Black Butte
5.2 miles round trip, difficult

Although from nearby I-5 a climb up Black Butte appears to demand a horrific scree struggle, in fact a groomed, occasionally rocky trail climbs 2000 feet to its summit, steadily bringing one to some of the most impressive perspectives of Shasta and the region.

TRAILHEAD

Drive 2.0 miles up Everitt Highway, to where the highway starts a long curve right, and turn left (W) onto a dirt road signed for Black Butte. After 0.1 mile turn right (N), and continue for 1.0 mile to a junction. Turn left (W) for 0.4 mile and then curve right (N), staying

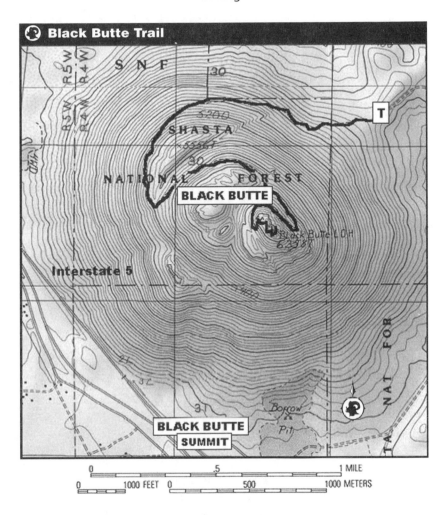

Black Butte Trail

on the main dirt road. This soon curves left (W) and after **1.2** miles you reach a junction where you turn left (S). This final leg curves right (W) and climbs very steeply to the trailhead, 5.3 miles from the start of the highway.

DESCRIPTION

This trail begins with a long, rising arc around Black Butte's north slopes, taking you across talus slopes scattered with white firs, ponderosa pines, Douglas-firs and squaw currant. Brilliantly colored lichens crust over many of the sharp gray blocks of dacite here. As you curve to the north and northwest sides of Black Butte, the hillocks of Shasta Valley come into view, and one can try to imagine the immensity of the landslide off of Shasta that created that bumpy terrain (see the "Geology" chapter). Beyond rises the symmetrical cone of Mt. McLoughlin, in Oregon.

As you work around to the west slopes of the butte, you see Mt. Eddy rising above I-5 and Strawberry Valley below, and to the southeast you see some of the Castle Crags as well as distant Lassen Peak. Now you cut back northeast through a secluded ravine, a gap between two of Black Butte's four overlapping cones. Along here the trail is at its rockiest, but better tread soon takes you from a red-fir grove to a "near-enough-to-touch" panorama of Mt. Shasta. Always in full view of Shasta now, you continue climbing around to Black Butte's east slopes, then cut back to the north, not far from the summit. Tighter switchbacks occupy your last quarter mile to the top, where all the panoramas you've seen come together in a breathtaking 360-degree view of the region.

Gumboot Saddle to Castle Crags on the Pacific Crest Trail

25.1 miles one way, moderate

Here is the longest stretch of unroaded trail in the Shasta region, and what a spectacular tour it delivers. From panoramic cruising along the Sacramento-Trinity divide down to hidden fringes of the Castle Crags, this section of the PCT looks over some of northern California's prime scenery. To hike the whole route most people will want to arrange a car shuttle and make a weekend of it. Fit hikers do complete it in a long day, however. This route also is popular for hikers starting from either direction and walking in as far as they wish, then retracing back to their trailhead.

TRAILHEADS

If you wish to leave a car at Castle Crags (which is 4400 feet lower than the Gumboot trailhead), you have two options. One is to arrange a spot within the Park with the Castle Crags State Park rangers, as overnight parking is not allowed at the Park's trailheads. The other is to leave it at the Soda Springs exit off I-5, 2 miles north of the Castle Crags–Castella turnoff. Park along the frontage road running below the east side of the freeway.

To reach Gumboot Saddle, from downtown Mount Shasta drive southwest over the Interstate and curve to a "T" at Old Stage Road. Turn left (south) and after **0.3** mile veer right on W. A. Barr road, toward Lake Siskiyou. Continue across the lake's dam and stay on this road as it curves west. Next, avoid a spur road to the left, and keep on the main road as it curves south and becomes Forest Rd. 26. Follow this up the canyon of the South Fork of the Sacramento River, and after about **9** miles keep right at the Gumboot Lake spur. Stay on the paved road as it switchbacks another **2.5** miles to the saddle, 18.5 miles from downtown Mount Shasta. From either trailhead it's smart to start hiking well stocked with water.

DESCRIPTION

From Gumboot Saddle begin trekking south on the PCT, rising gradually, and soon you'll arc into another saddle. This is the PCT's manner along this divide: garland-style traversing from saddle to saddle. At brief turns onto the east-facing side around small crags, you get views over the Gumboot lakes, and beyond to Mt. Shasta. This side drains to the Sacramento River and San Francisco Bay. On the west side arcs you stride where snow melt heads for the Trinity River and eventually the Klamath River estuary. Just over a mile of divide-cruising brings you to a steady traverse of a

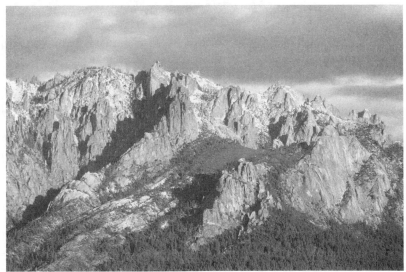

Castle Crags

granitic talus slope, where morning light displays fine views of the Trinity Alps, about 15 miles distant.

This traverse ends at a major saddle and a view over Seven Lakes Basin, about 500 feet below. Along this saddle a rough path runs south to an eroding and rarely used jeep trail that crosses the crest and drops east to the lakes. The PCT immediately turns east at the crest, starting you on your commitment to the Sacramento

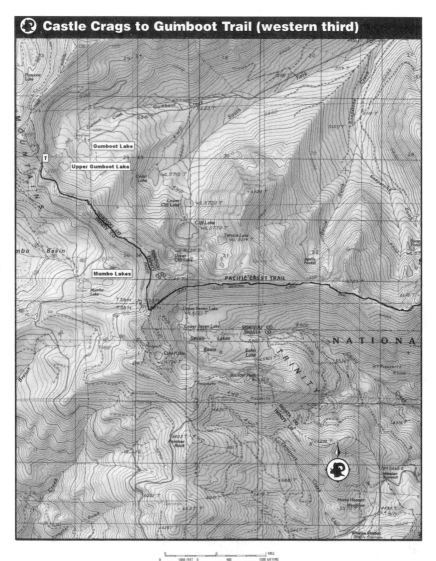

headwaters with a long and panoramic traverse. From rocky and brushy slopes you look down on the indigo Seven Lakes, and then across to the craggy facets of Boulder Peak lifting right out of Echo Lake.

The pleasant walking continues onto a low point in the spine between Castle Creek and the Sacramento's South Fork, where the prospects encompass a broad domain. From Lassen Peak far to the

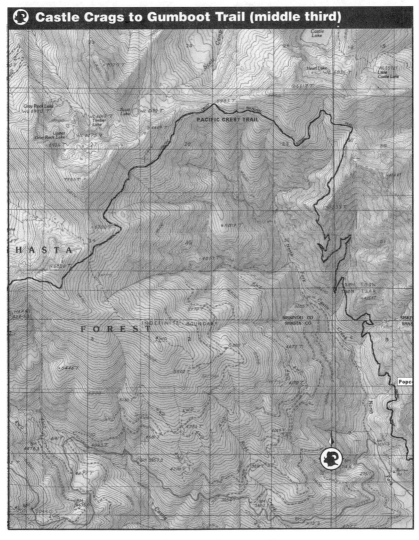

Castle Crags to Gumboot Trail (middle third)

southeast, to Shasta in the northeast, and around to ruddy Mt. Eddy almost due north, the views from this spot (5 miles from the trailhead) make a worthwhile destination for dayhikers.

Next you hike an imperceptible rise to a spur, then turn north and descend through a shady forest of red fir and white fir. These woods break open at another spur, where you get your last view of

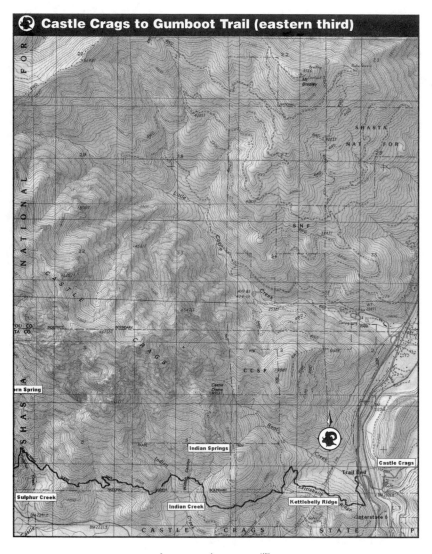

Mt. Shasta and your first view of the Castle Crags. This point, 7 miles from the trailhead, makes another excellent goal for round-trip dayhikers, as this western vista shows many domes and turrets that highway travelers can never know. Yet even this vista only hints at the full extent of Castle Crags' fantastic uplift.

A short distance north from this viewpoint is a small, rocky bench, which cups a shallow, ephemeral pool into early summer. Here you have begun a broad arc around the head of the North Fork of Castle Creek. Steady traversing with modest rises and descents takes you across verdant slopes of manzanita, huckleberry oak and chinquapin, greenery rich with wildflowers in early season. Behind you to the south, the Grey Rocks rise, a meta-volcanic forebear of the granitic Castle Crags.

A couple of miles from your initial Crag view you meet the lowest saddle in the ridgeline you have been contouring below, a notch where small white firs and mountain hemlocks spill over from adjacent north-facing slopes. In 0.75 mile more to the west, your path crosses a freshet that nourishes a crowd of insectivorous pitcher plants. After midsummer this spring may be the first water across the trail since the trailhead (9.8 miles), and the only water to come for another few miles. In dry years even this may not issue enough to fill a bottle. Contouring continues into a larger drainage that nevertheless runs with water only into midsummer. As you leave this arroyo, you start descending, reaching in 0.5 mile a pass with nice but dry camping among stately white firs.

Now your trail veers southwest off the pass to dramatically change in character, for you start in earnest a 2200-foot descent. The first leg slants down slopes where chinquapin and huckleberry oak grow in some places thick into the path's corridor. The brush relents as you break onto rockier ground and descend past solitary knobcone and sugar pines. Soon you begin some well-constructed switchbacks that lead you south back and forth down and across the face of a rocky prow, giving you closer vistas of dramatic Crag walls. Keen eyes will spot along here an unusual arch of granite among the parapets above.

This upper reach of the Crags was the final hideout for braves of the Wintun tribe. Miners, loggers and Army harassment had pushed the Indians to this rugged sanctuary, and in 1855 the Wintun's last stand was here. Joaquin Miller, a miner and writer usually sympathetic to Indians, was wounded in this battle. He finessed this incident into a claim to heroism in the famous Modoc War, and he entertained packed houses in Europe with this fable.

49

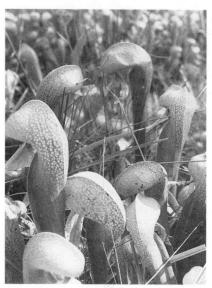

Pitcher plant, or Darlingtonia

To this day a legend persists that the Wintun stashed a fortune in gold somewhere among the Crags.

Soon a long switchback takes you way back to near the narrow trough of a seasonal creek, and then you reverse again into forest, now thicker with Douglas-firs, ponderosa pines and oaks. Once more you switchback to near the streambed, and then make a weaving descent to cross the drainage where it probably carries water throughout most years. Here in the shade of dense Oregon oaks one could bivouac.

Now the PCT contours into the next drainage east, where outlying knobs and walls loom intimate, and more splintery towers march away up rugged glens. You switchback again, descend along a sandy spur, and then cut back across and out of the seasonally watered ravine. Then you traverse south and come to Popcorn Spring. This generally reliable fount dribbles under dense oak and Douglas-fir shade. Contouring from here continues south to a junction with the "Dog Trail," an unsigned path that descends to the logging road along the North Fork of Castle Creek. It allows dog owners to access or exit the PCT by circumventing Castle Crags State Park, where dogs are not allowed. From the junction, continue around a knob of rusty peridotite and get some great views of the magnificent walls around Battle Mountain, one of the biggest and steepest brows in the Crags. Now you need to keep an eye out for poison oak as the trail switchbacks past a small landslide down to Sulphur Creek.

The route then turns a spur to cross Sulphur Creek's east fork, another fairly reliable stream. Dense Douglas-fir and incense-cedar forest shades the traversing trail for another 0.75 mile to a spur with a nice view out to Grey Rocks. Switchbacks then descend past knobcone pines to resume a traverse to Dump Creek. Across this creek an unsigned trail descends south, but keep contouring to a pair of switchbacks that work up to a slightly higher traverse. This traverse wends in and out of many gullies and takes you into Castle Crags State Park, where camping is allowed only at the roadside campgrounds. Now cruising through brushier terrain, you get new perspectives of the Crags above before descending to Indian Creek. Back in shade that would be quite welcome on a midsummer afternoon, the trail curves into Wintun Canyon and then across the twin eastern forks of Indian Creek.

The traversing continues around a ridge, past the last good view of the Castle Crags, and soon crosses the first of the State Park's well-groomed paths, the Bob's Hat Trail. If you left a car near the Park's headquarters, you'll want to descend Bob's Hat Trail to the nearby road and continue on pavement for not quite a mile to finish your hike. If you parked at I-5, from the Bob's Hat junction, hike east a quarter mile, then start descending under a variety of oaks and ponderosa pines to the level crest of Kettlebelly Ridge and an intersection. The Castle Dome Trail runs east-west along this ridgecrest, while the PCT/Root Creek Trail turns north. Follow this, but you will soon leave the Root Creek Trail on its contour and veer downhill on the PCT. Three short switchbacks reverse south to cross under interstate power lines, and then turn east across the shady north slopes of Kettlebelly Ridge. This traverse ends just shy of the ridge's prow, where the Kettlebelly Trail continues south, and where you cut back north for the last half-mile descent to I-5. Now on an old roadbed, you hike to the freeway, and turn through the underpass to meet your car.

Parks Creek Summit to Deadfall Lakes and Gumboot Saddle on the Pacific Crest Trail

13.6 miles one way, moderate

This segment of the PCT follows the northernmost reach of the open, subalpine divide between the Trinity and Sacramento rivers. Its top-of-the-world routing curves by a number of serene lakes tucked under the divide, making it a prime tour for an overnight or a leisurely three-day backpack. Many dayhikers and overnighters enjoy a round-trip stint to any of a few nice destinations along this stretch of PCT, or with a car shuttle one can hike the complete route one-way.

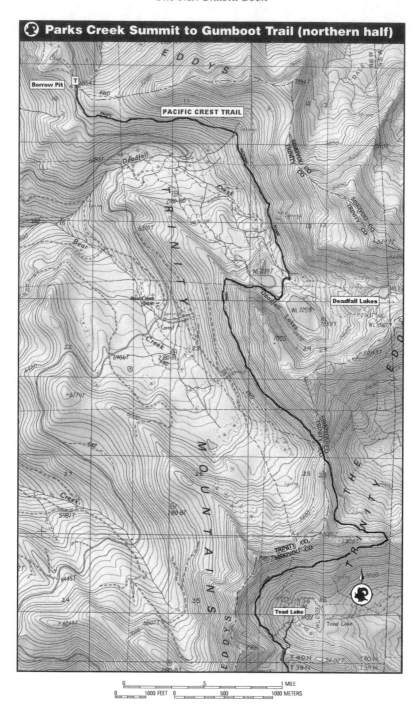

Parks Creek Summit to Gumboot Trail (northern half)

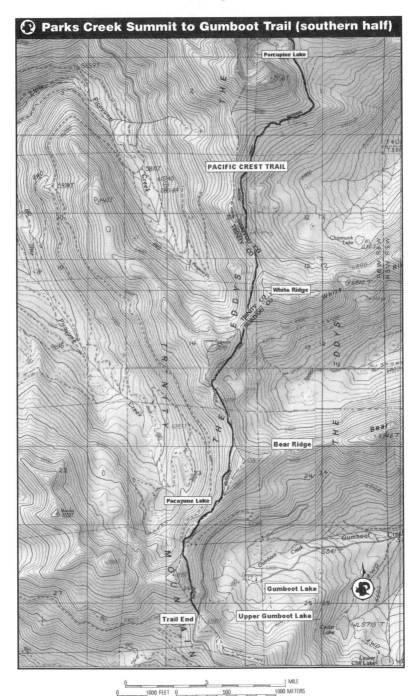

Parks Creek Summit to Gumboot Trail (southern half)

Porcupine Lake

PACIFIC CREST TRAIL

White Ridge

Bear Ridge

Pacayune Lake

Gumboot Lake

Trail End

Upper Gumboot Lake

TRAILHEADS

The north end of this route starts at Parks Creek Summit. To get there, drive north on I-5 3.4 miles past the Weed turnoff and take the Edgewood-Gazelle exit. Turn southwest under the freeway to a T, and take the right (NW) fork. After 0.4 mile turn left (SW) onto Stewart Springs Road–Forest Road 17. Keep right on this road after 3.9 miles; as it gets steeper, stay on paved Road 17 to the summit, 12.9 miles from the Stewart Springs turnoff.

To reach Gumboot Saddle, from downtown Mount Shasta drive southwest over the Interstate and curve to a "T" at Old Stage Road. Turn left (south) and after 0.3 mile veer right on W. A. Barr road, toward Lake Siskiyou. Continue across the lake's dam and stay on this road as it curves west. Next, avoid a spur road to the left, and keep on the main road as it curves south and becomes Forest Rd. 26. Follow this up the canyon of the South Fork of the Sacramento River, and after about 9 miles keep right at the Gumboot Lake spur. Stay on the paved road as it switchbacks another 2.5 miles to the saddle, 18.5 miles from downtown Mount Shasta.

DESCRIPTION

From Parks Creek Summit you strike southeast on the well-groomed Pacific Crest Trail, noting right away a diversity of conifers that only these Trinity Mountains hold. In contouring one long slope, you pass beneath Jeffrey pines, red firs, white firs, Douglas-firs, western white pines and lodgepole pines. Before too long you emerge onto flowery glades where year-round springs run across the trail, and the views open west to the Scott Mountains. Just ahead, 2.1 miles from the car, you reach Deadfall Creek and intersect the modern end of the Sisson-Callahan Trail. This heads southwest past upper Deadfall Lake.

Take the PCT south to near the northwest corner of this pretty lake, which has excellent and popular campsites near its west and east shores, and reflections of russet Mt. Eddy in its waters. Lower Deadfall Lake is also accessible below the trail, and it offers a peaceful alternative camp when a holiday weekend brings many to seek this country.

The PCT route turns northeast away from the lake and traverses a granitic talus slope, then enters red-fir woods and turns south around a ridgeline. Continued forest hiking takes you to an ancient and unusual type of bedrock, peridotite. The views open up as you angle through a pass, where Mt. Shasta rises into domination. Here you cross the original Sisson-Callahan Trail. This historic track is still obvious descending east from this pass, but in the basin below the old path disappears. To the west the trail still can be followed down to logging roads along Bear Creek.

Peridotite

This russet-and-mustard colored stone is thought to be a relic of the earth's mantle extruded from an ancient ocean floor. Rafted along by millions of years of geologic turmoil, the peridotite now rests among newer rock formations, and in North America it is nowhere common except here in the Klamath-Trinity Mountains. Its ultramafic (high magnesium and iron) mineral content discourages tree growth, so peridotite areas usually appear somewhat barren, with stunted vegetation.

Continue on the PCT through the pass, and south onto east-facing slopes, where foxtail pines make a strong effort on the peridotite. Open, easy walking continues past bizarre, crusty-banded outcrops and patches of sulphur flower and gilia, and up to another saddle. Here you find a distant panorama past the Castle Crags. The sky-walk next cuts west and starts descending into fir forest to round the cirque of Toad Lake, generally visible below. Four hundred feet above the lake's northwest corner you meet an old trail that's no longer traceable down to the lake. The well-aimed PCT arcs south to just below the cirque's exit saddle, from where an old set of steep switchbacks can be followed down to the lake. Quiet campsites await around its shores.

From the exit saddle, hike south onto gentle ground and descend some along an old moraine with head-high firs and hemlocks. Along this section watch for an unmarked trail branching west to weave uphill; this is the path to Porcupine Lake, just five minutes away. Diorite cliffs, fir and hemlock stands, and clear, chilly water make this lake reminiscent of the northern High Sierra. The staccato of kingfishers rings over these waters, and excellent campsites are found off its east and north shores. Overnighters from Gumboot Saddle often make this their destination, 3.9 miles from the trailhead.

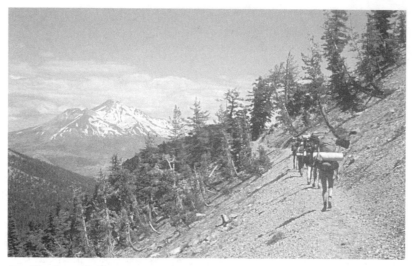

Pacific Crest Trail

From the Porcupine turnoff, continue south on a rocky contour, rounding a spur at an excellent view of Mt. Shasta. Next, traverse the head of a broad basin where the lowing of grazing cattle often calls through the meadows. Near the south end of this traverse you pass above a spring surrounded by Darlingtonia, or pitcher plant. This cobra-shaped carnivore lures insects into its throat with a musty-sweet aroma, then traps them with sticky, down-pointing hairs. Symbiotic bacteria and invertebrates then start taking in the bugs, and the plant enjoys the final digestion of nutrients. Darlingtonia lives only in this region, and it seems to find advantage on soggy and ultramafic substrates.

You hike south out of this basin to another excellent vista east, then cross the divide and get a whole new view west to the Trinity Alps. Now on a rise of white granite, you pass the Picayune Trail descending to logging roads along Little Picayune Creek. You swing back across the divide for a view of Lassen Peak, then back to the west side again to walk under western white pines and white firs, getting glimpses of Picayune Lake not far below. The panoramic views invite you to pause as you return to rust-toned peridotite ground and gently descend, swinging from one saddle to two more saddles. At the last low point you cross a dirt road and keep hiking south. From a final good view of Shasta, the trail veers to make a switchback down to Gumboot Saddle, where you arrive at a small parking lot and the road from Lake Siskiyou.

Deadfall Lakes and Mt. Eddy Climb, on the Sisson-Callahan Trail

12.2 miles one way, difficult

Running from subalpine lakes and meadows to lowland transition forest and chaparral, this historical trail is an introduction to the botanically rich Trinity Mountains. It also offers a side trip to the top of Mt. Eddy, where perhaps the most overwhelming view of Mt. Shasta awaits. The hike to here, or just to the Deadfall Lakes and back, is the most popular segment of this trail.

As a route, the Sisson-Callahan dates back probably to Indians, and certainly to trappers, prospectors and cattlemen of the mid-1800s. The Forest Service constructed it in 1911, to link Forest Headquarters in Sisson (Mount Shasta) with Callahan. The west half of the trail, beyond the Trinity-Sacramento divide, is traceable but largely masked by logging and mining roads. However, the east half, described here, passes through nearly uninterrupted backcountry, and has been designated a National Recreation Trail.

As described here, the hike starts from Parks Creek Summit on the Pacific Crest Trail, and then takes the relocated Sisson-Callahan route over Deadfall Summit and down the north fork of the Sacramento River to the eastern trailhead near Lake Siskiyou. To hike its entirety you either need to arrange a car shuttle or to plan a long round trip—too long for most hikers in one day. For the full hike, most people prefer to start at higher Parks Creek Summit, for a net descent of 3200 feet to the eastern trailhead.

TRAILHEADS

To reach Parks Creek Summit, drive north on I-5 **3.4** miles past the Weed turnoff and take the Edgewood-Gazelle exit. Turn southwest under the freeway to a T, and take the right (NW) fork. After **0.4** mile turn left (SW) onto Stewart Springs Road–Forest Road 17. Keep right on this road after **3.9** miles; as it gets steeper, stay on paved Road 17 to the summit, 12.9 miles from the Stewart Springs turnoff.

To get to the eastern trailhead, from downtown Mount Shasta cross I-5 at the main Mount Shasta exit and continue southwest to a T at Old Stage Road. Turn left (NW) and soon veer right onto W.A. Barr Road, toward Lake Siskiyou. A mile from the Old Stage turnoff, turn right onto North Shore Road 40N27. Drive along the north shore of Lake Siskiyou, keeping left at the only minor fork, and park near where the road ends at the North Fork of the Sacramento River. From here the trail follows an old roadbed that heads up the opposite side of the river.

DESCRIPTION

From Parks Creek Summit you strike southeast on the well-groomed Pacific Crest Trail, noting right away a diversity of conifers that only these Trinity Mountains hold. In contouring one long slope, you pass beneath Jeffrey pines, red firs, white firs, Douglas-firs, western white pines and lodgepole pines. Before too long you emerge onto flowery glades where year-round springs run across the trail, and the views open west to the Scott Mountains. Just ahead, 2.1 miles from the car, you reach Deadfall Creek and meet the Deadfall Trail, now also the modern end of the Sisson-Callahan Trail.

Those who want to camp, swim, fish or just visit the largest and best of the Deadfall Lakes will want to continue on the PCT a minute farther, cross the outlet stream and turn uphill to find the lake nearby. The Sisson-Callahan route turns southeast, up another shallow drainage.

Now you enjoy meadows, forest and high views ahead to Mt. Eddy on a steady climb, which before long steepens up a shallow ravine. Soon you reach a bench containing one of the smaller Deadfall lakes, and you circle along its west shore, eyeing the waters for the trout that make this basin a favorite with anglers. Next, hop a stream and rise to a slightly higher bench that cups a larger lake, a subalpine gem reflecting the craggy ochre face of Mt. Eddy. After cruising along the meadowy south shore of this lake, you start the final climb to Deadfall Summit.

A single switchback takes you south out of the last lake's small cirque and up through one of the most diverse stands of conifers you'll ever see; on these slopes grow red fir, white fir, lodgepole pine, western white pine, whitebark pine and foxtail pine. It's thought that such diversity exists because these Trinity mountains have maintained a stable-climate refuge for many different plant species. Over recent millennia, alternating glaciations and droughts around the West have created stresses for many species, and as a moist semi-coastal range having only small glaciers, the Klamath-Trinitys have kept a steadier climate. Plants driven from the south during droughts have found moist refuge here, and

Mt. Eddy Ascent

2.8 miles round trip, 1000-foot gain

Although no trail junction to Mt. Eddy is obvious from the Sisson-Callahan Trail, it's not hard to leave the latter track and find the old trail built to service the now-abandoned lookout atop Mt. Eddy. About 100 yards southeast of Deadfall Summit, head east-northeast on a gradually ascending traverse. In about 0.1 mile you should pick up the trail near the first switchback. If not, head more directly upslope, and you'll soon come across a very clear track.

The first few switchbacks climb through a surprisingly dense stand of foxtail pine, an uncommon relative of the bristlecone pine, which grows only in these mountains, and in the southern Sierra. The switchbacks touch the Trinity-Shasta divide a couple of times, and then one long switchback cuts back east onto slopes where scattered whitebark pines gradually replace the foxtails. Now a steady bank of tighter switchbacks climbs into the rocky alpine realm of the hulsea, penstemon, and krummholz whitebarks.

The toil to the summit rewards one with a stunning view of Mt. Shasta. Perhaps from no other place can one feel so intensely the overwhelming immensity of Shasta. Atop Mt. Eddy a vestigial lookout still stands, though it was abandoned in 1931.

plants pushed down from the north have found refuge from advancing glaciers.

The short final climb to Deadfall Summit gives you a distant view west beyond the Deadfall basin over the subalpine ridge country of Scott Mountain and over much of the rest of the Trinity River country. You cross the pass into the Sacramento River watershed, and about 100 yards southeast of the crest you come to a cairn, which marks the spot where those who want to climb Mt. Eddy will branch north.

Continuing on the Sisson-Callahan Trail, you start a steep descent south off Deadfall Summit, braking through duff down into a meadowy realm of fir and chinquapin. Before too long switchbacks ease the grade, and on the easternmost of these hairpins you come within 100 yards of a gushing spring, which, along

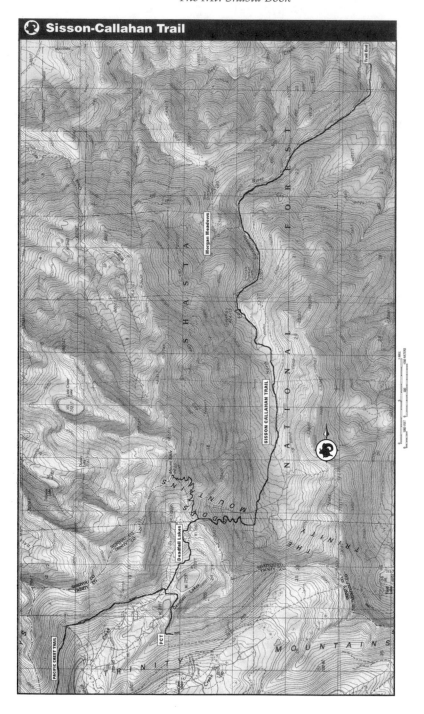

with springs on Mt. Shasta, is one of the sources of the Sacramento River. Depression-era license plates high on the trees mark your trail as an old snow-survey route, and eventually you pass near the remains of the surveyor's old cabin, which burned down in 2003.

Turning southeast here, you continue on a more gradually descending traverse. Here you might notice the faint trail that runs west back over the divide. This is the original Sisson-Callahan track. The newer eastbound trail becomes a bit obscure also, but numerous tree blazes guide you on a continued downhill traverse to the North Fork of the Sacramento, at which point there is a quiet stream with stones you can hop across. Here another old trail heads southwest to climb over to the Middle Fork drainage, and you continue east along the Sacramento, ambling through glades and groves of white fir, lodgepole pine and surprisingly large incense-cedars. As you reach leveler, soggier ground the glades become richer with brodiaea, potentilla, columbine and yarrow, allowing broader views to ridgelines that rim the valley with peridotite.

At one meadow the grasses have partly overgrown the trail, and you'll want to continue on a straight course across the north side of this meadow to find a dry, rocky creekbed that after a short distance leads into distinct trail. Paralleling the North Fork of the Sacramento, this gentle descent continues for another 0.5 mile, to where a couple of switchbacks start the drop out of the once-glaciated high country into the river's lower canyon. The switchbacks empty onto an old roadbed, which you follow for nearly 0.5 mile before coming to a sisson-callahan trail marker on the north edge of the road. At this post, unfortunately easy to miss without a watchful eye, you drop off the road and start a steady descent along the now-tumbling Sacramento River.

Under sugar pines, Jeffrey pines and Douglas-firs, the trail follows the river canyon's curve to the southeast, passing an old jeep road that climbs south, and then descending on a couple of small switchbacks. Continue descending past a waterfall and into warmer climes, where beargrass, pipsissiwa, paintbrush, Shasta lily and azalea catch your eye. As you descend farther, breaks in the forest let you look back for a last glimpse at the eastern summits of Mt. Eddy. Eventually the trail runs onto an old roadbed, which takes you across a tributary creek and curves east down to the old crossing of the main river. Here you can hop rocks or perhaps wet your feet to ford to the eastern trailhead, on North Shore Road.

Pluto Cave

0.5 mile to 1 mile (length of the cave), easy

Many volcanic regions have what are called lava tubes, caves formed when the outer surface of a lava flow cools and congeals, but the still-molten core flows on and evacuates the congealed shell. A number of lava tubes are found around Shasta, some of which are a mile or more long, and the most famous is Pluto Cave.

Venturing into this large cave should not be taken lightly. The depths of Pluto Cave are eternally dark, so take at least two working flashlights; headlamps are better, to keep your hands free. The temperature inside remains a cool 50°F year-round, so bring warm clothes. The way is occasionally quite rocky, so wear sturdy footgear and choose your steps carefully. Finally, don't go alone. While the seriousness of somehow getting lost in the cave should not be overlooked, for those who are careful the eerie experience of advancing into a seemingly infinite blackness is unforgettable.

TRAILHEAD

From the Weed stoplight, drive northeast on Hwy. 97 for **10.6** miles to County Road A12. On it go northwest **3.3** miles, and at the end of a long, gentle downgrade turn left (W) onto a dirt road. As of 2005, signs point out this turnoff. Drive west and southwest on this road for about **0.5** mile to the trailhead near the entrance to the cave.

DESCRIPTION

The track forks at a large juniper tree and either fork will take you to the cave. If you walk west-southwest on the right-hand fork for about a quarter mile, you follow spray-painted rocks and come to a large depression in the ground; this is the vague beginning of Pluto Cave. Walk right (N) a short distance along the rim of the depression to a path descending into it. Certain areas of the cave have blocks hanging down from the ceiling, and for this reason some cavers recommend wearing a helmet to protect against head bumps. There can be seasonal closures of Pluto Cave to protect nesting bats. Information on current conditions of the cave and possible seasonal closures may be obtained from the Goosenest Ranger Station, (530) 398-4391.

If you walk southwest on the left-hand fork, after about a quarter mile you come onto a well-graded cinder road. Walk west

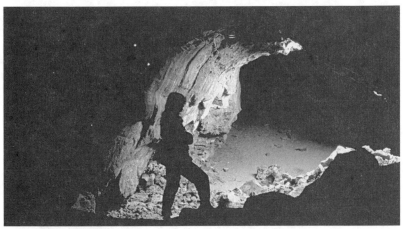

Inside Pluto Cave

down this for a short distance to a mound of blocks. Among these blocks is the more distant entrance to the cave. Walk north into the entrance and soon you'll come to an opening, the depression mentioned in the other road fork. A path runs northwest through the surprisingly lush floor of the depression, leading you to the depths of Pluto Cave.

The dusty path leads between boulders into growing darkness. But this is only a preliminary darkness, for you soon come underneath some large gaps in the 20 foot-high ceiling of the cave. Some graffiti on the walls date to the early 20th century, and it's interesting to contrast the careful hand of the earlier adventurers with today's spray-painted scrawls. After a couple hundred yards you pass the last light, and descend into absolute darkness. A rocky, dusty track leads on, with occasional spots where you have to scramble across boulders. The way continues farther than most are inclined to venture—at least a mile.

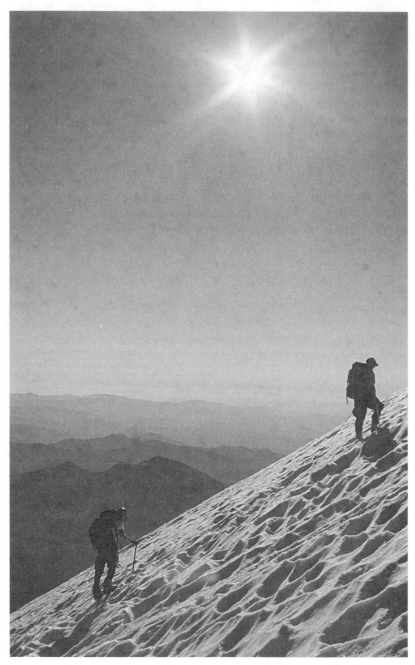

Climbers on the Hotlum-Bolam Ridge

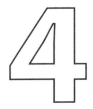

CLIMBING

THE HIGH MOUNTAINS have a special allure for those who go up into the cirques and high meadows, and onto the arêtes and peaks. Life itself seems more sparkling as the mountains become our window to a richer, clearer reality. The variety of our mountain experiences can be endless: There are different "paths" to be followed in climbing mountains—different personal paths as well as different routes on the peaks.

Although a great mountain like Shasta has special rewards for those who venture onto it, life on the heights is not always easy, and our goals may be hard to achieve. Certainly even the best mountaineers and other outdoorsmen have known discomfort, difficulty and even fear. In fact, knowledge and understanding of adversity are what set the seasoned adventurer apart from those with less experience.

The enjoyment, challenge and satisfaction of climbing should always be tempered with concern for safety. This book can help you discover some wonderful, exciting places on Mt. Shasta, but it's no substitute for experience, careful preparations and good judgment. You are responsible for your own safety. To ensure it, you must get proper mountaineering training and then exercise caution and common sense based on that training plus experience. Many outdoor organizations and clubs, and college and university recreation programs, have mountaineering courses. These courses are a good way to learn climbing from experienced climbers.

Mt. Shasta shows many changes and many moods over the seasons. A climb up the John Muir/Avalanche Gulch route during the long, calm days of early summer is usually sublime. The same climb during winter can be very serious and difficult. During ample snow years many of the northside and eastside routes remain in excellent condition with hard snow throughout the summer and fall. However, in drier years, and generally by autumn of normal years, they can become glassy ice. We recommend that you always check weather and snow conditions before starting a hike or a climb. We also urge you to be honest with yourself and your climbing partners regarding your goals, experience, gear requirements, and even your mind-set. Mountains must be met on their own terms. Therefore, take responsibility for your judgment, actions and welfare.

Many emergencies and fatalities have occurred on Mt. Shasta, and rescue is often lengthy, dangerous and uncertain. Rescues may be delayed by unfavorable weather, unavailability of helicopters able to fly in the thin air of the upper altitudes, hazards to rescuers and other problems.

The Siskiyou County Sheriff's Department is responsible for coordinating rescue efforts on Mt. Shasta, but unless an accident is known to have happened, they will not take action until *after* your expected return date has passed. Your wilderness permit information can be utilized for rescue purposes, but it is not a rescuer's document and there is no sign-out.

We've chosen what we think are the finest routes on Mt. Shasta, along with some selected variations. The route descriptions are fairly general—partly because the mountain is never quite the same from season to season, and partly so as not to deprive you of a sense of adventure. Many of the routes do not require a rope, but most require ice ax and crampons, and knowledge of their use. Other routes require more experience, specialized equipment, glacier training and crevasse rescue knowledge. Some of the summit routes are quite long if started from base camp, so we've mentioned some high camps to break the climb into shorter days, if you choose. The climbing routes are listed clockwise around the mountain beginning on the southwest side at the historic John Muir/Avalanche Gulch climb.

DIFFICULTY RATINGS

Until very recently there was no rating system in North America that would accurately apply to climbs on alpine peaks such as Mt. Shasta. Thus, the authors of this book developed an ad-hoc D1-3 rating system (below) to apply only on Mt. Shasta, showing the relative difficulty among the peak's routes. However, within the last few years North American alpine climbers have begun to apply the increasingly universal French system of alpine grades. As interpreted in North America, this system apprises all the challenges of a mountain route—from scale and amount of technical climbing to general climate and descent options, as follows:

F　**(Facil—easy)**
PD　**(Peu Difficil—somewhat difficult)**
AD　**(Assez Difficil—fairly difficult)**
D　**(Difficile—difficult)**
TD　**(Trés Difficile—very difficult)**
ED　**(Extrémenent Difficile—extremely difficult)**

The climbs on Mt. Shasta have substantial scale, but the easiest ones require little technical climbing, so they are rated D1, or F, "easy." The most difficult routes require a reasonable degree of technical climbing, and are rated D3, or AD. These ratings of course are subjective, and they reflect typical climbing conditions. In storm or icy conditions, for instance, a climb can be more difficult than the rating implies.

Dl, or F: 3rd class. Moderate terrain and moderate conditions, either rock or snow, requiring proper footwear, ice ax and crampons. A rope is generally not needed, but may be taken in reserve for less experienced members.

　　Examples:　R 1　　John Muir/Avalanche Gulch
　　　　　　　　R 15　　Clear Creek

D2, or PD: 4th class. A rope is necessary for belaying and protection but the climbing is not very difficult. Traveling on crevassed glaciers may be necessary, but the terrain and route finding are moderate.

　　Examples:　R 5　　Casaval Ridge
　　　　　　　　R 8　　Bolam Glacier

D3, or AD: Similar to 5th class. Difficult ice and snow or rock requiring specialized equipment and advanced technique. The glaciers may have steep icefalls, many crevasses and difficult route finding.

　　Example:　R 11　　Hotlum Glacier

An Alpine Climbing Primer for Mt. Shasta

Any climb of Shasta is a strenuous endeavor into high alpine terrain, where the dynamics of snow, ice, rock and sky determine how—or if—one should climb. Mt. Shasta is many people's first foray into such elemental heights. Unfortunately, accidents and even fatalities continue, most of which could have been avoided with a bit more alpine savviness. Here are some basic rules of thumb to bear in mind when attempting a Shasta climb:

Anyone climbing any route on Mt. Shasta needs to be competent with an ice ax and crampons on moderately steep slopes. These tools and skills open up Shasta's best surface for going up—snow, frozen and firm.

The mountain is in prime shape in early summer, and it is best climbed with a pre-dawn start and a commitment to be back down no later than early afternoon. In the heat later in the day, snow can get swampy and slow for travel, and snowbridges over crevasses, moats and bergschrunds are more likely to collapse underfoot. Worse, melting temperatures make rockfall more likely. In addition to timing your climb to the conditions, minimize your exposure to rockfall by adjusting your route to avoid ravines that funnel tumbling stones.

As the summer progresses and the snow retreats, conditions become more difficult because more rock is exposed, which takes more effort to climb and opens up more possible rockfall, In addition, late summer snow often consolidates into glassy ice, an especially common problem on the north-side routes. If you are unfamiliar with the techniques to handle hard ice, the high slopes on Shasta are not the place to experiment.

Whatever the season, you need good weather to climb Mt. Shasta. Rest assured that any foul weather will be amplified dramatically high on the peak, so check the forecast before you decide to climb.

Shasta's great vertical relief demands a substantial level of fitness, including an awareness of pacing, refueling, and an understanding of how the thin air of high altitude affects your performance. If your pace slows to a crawl and you don't recover after a rest, you are either exhausted, dehydrated, hungry, cold, or suffering from the altitude—or all of the above—and you should retreat.

Coming down is easier when the snow has softened, but not so much that it's sloppy. Descent normally goes much faster than ascent, but going down is at least as hazardous as going up, because this is when a party is most tired, and when snow, rockfall, and weather conditions are more likely to worsen.

Routefinding also can be more difficult on the way down, so as you climb up take frequent looks down to memorize your route back. When there's an open and familiar snow slope to descend, it can be safe to follow an old Shasta tradition and glissade, either on your boot soles or on your bum. Glissading can be a superb way to get down fast and fun, but it has also been the initiation of many accidents on Shasta. Unwary climbers set off into a thrilling ride, but then slide into unexpected ice, sail into unexpected crevasses, accelerate beyond their ability to brake, or catch their crampons. Glissade only with an ice ax and a practiced ability to stop with it, and only when you know the slope below is continuous snow with no ice, rocks or crevasses. And always take off your crampons first.

If the whole endeavor of climbing Shasta seems enticing but you're not quite sure you're up for it on your own, a variety of guide services are available.

If we know how to listen, a mountain like Shasta tells us when, where and how it can be climbed. All the hazards are manageable, and really, it's the experience of working through challenges that makes a climb rewarding, no?

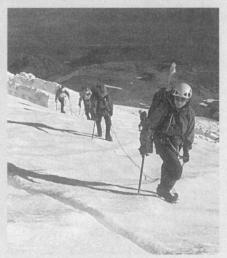

Hotlum Glacier Climb

CHRIS CARR/SHASTA MOUNTAIN GUIDES

Times listed are conservative averages for round trip from base camp. Actual time can vary greatly due to weather, snow and ice conditions, strength of party and other reasons. Times are indicated in days and fractions thereof.

On popular climbing routes, human waste has become a problem on high slopes where it cannot decompose and where people depend on snowmelt for water. Therefore the Forest Service requires all climbers and hikers to pack out their waste. At their office and at the trailheads they offer free zip-lock packets with paper bags and kitty litter. Some climbers use kayakers' "dry bags" to ensure a bombproof carry out. In any case, the inner bags can then be disposed of in the special containers at the trailheads.

Access to the trailheads is described in detail in the "Hiking" chapter. The best base-camp and high-camp locations are indicated in the route descriptions.

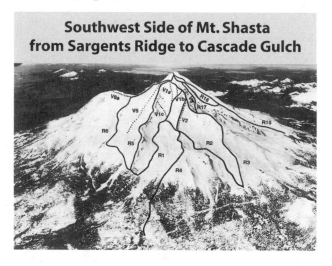

Southwest Side of Mt. Shasta from Sargents Ridge to Cascade Gulch

---

Route 1 **TRADITIONAL JOHN MUIR/ AVALANCHE GULCH**

DIFFICULTY: 1 (F)

ACCESS: Everitt Memorial Highway via Bunny Flat or Sand Flat

CAMPSITES: Horse Camp, Helen Lake, Sand Flat, Bunny Flat

TIME: 1 day

First Ascent

When General John C. Fremont journeyed past the east side of Mt. Shasta in 1846, he wrote that the mountain appeared to be "... nearly the height of Mont Blanc and unclimbable." Eight years later, on August 14, 1854, Elias D. Pierce of nearby Yreka led a group of seven friends up Shasta's southwest flank, accomplishing the first ascent. They marked the occasion by planting a large American flag at the summit. Pierce's success was not believed by the doubting public, who still thought Mt. Shasta was impossible to climb. Pierce therefore organized a second climb to prove his claims, and on September 19, 1854, nine climbers, led by Pierce, stood on Shasta's summit. Pierce succinctly remarked after his second successful climb:

There was no longer any doubt of the accessibility of the summit of Shasta Butte; although should one stand at its base and view its rugged form and towering peak, they would readily pronounce its ascent impossible.

The veil of impossibility had been lifted from Mt. Shasta, and other ascents quickly followed Pierce's two climbs. From 1854 to 1856 no less than 40 people (five women and 35 men) ascended the mountain. The first woman to climb Mt. Shasta was Olive Paddock Eddy, for whom nearby Mt. Eddy is named. She made several later ascents, and for many years held the record of most ascents of Shasta.

This was the route of the first recorded ascent of Mt. Shasta, by Captain E.D. Pierce in 1854, and is by far the most popular climbing route today. In the early days, before improved roads and all-weather highways, a climb began on horseback in Strawberry Valley in the town of Sisson. In those days guides and outfitters led their parties to timberline near the site of the present-day Sierra Club Foundation cabin at Horse Camp. Here, meadows provided forage and water for the horses while the party climbed.

Over the years increased use of this area brought improvement of the trail, construction of Olberman's Causeway, and establishment of campsites. Nevertheless, Horse Camp is still remarkably much like it was a century ago. There is still the gathering and the camaraderie of climbers from the world over, a summer custodian is in residence at

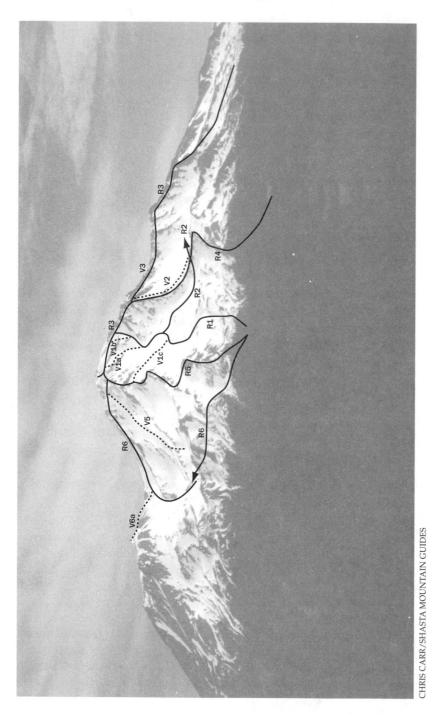

CHRIS CARR/SHASTA MOUNTAIN GUIDES

the cabin to help the first-time visitor, and the evenings are still the catalysts of tall tales. From the stone benches lining the rear wall of the cabin, you can see the panorama and many features of this climbing route. This is a wonderful base camp for one's first climb on Mt. Shasta.

From the Sierra Club Foundation cabin to the summit is only 4.1 miles, but over 6000 vertical feet! From a viewpoint just behind the cabin, the foreground vista (and the beginning of the climb) can be divided into three areas, from left to right: The climber's gully, the middle moraines and Avalanche Gulch. Olberman's Causeway, laboriously built of huge, flat stones by the cabin's first custodian, Mac Olberman, begins just a few feet behind the cabin and heads you in the proper direction.

You follow the causeway as it leads toward the peak. (When the causeway is still covered with snow, ascend the broad, main drainage behind the cabin.) Continue up the long climber's gully, which curves left, then straightens and opens up to a broad area of gentle flats and rock moraine. You are now at the left (W) of the huge, open drainage called Avalanche Gulch. Ascend moderate slopes upward to a flat area at 10,400 feet known as Helen Lake. You can also reach Helen Lake by ascending the morainal hills, just right (E) of the climber's gully. This line is a little more direct, but also steeper in places. Conditions at the time will dictate the best choice; consolidated snow is always easier climbing than loose talus. Few climbers use Avalanche Gulch proper as a means of ascent to Helen Lake, but it's often an excellent ski descent route.

Helen Lake was named in 1924 when Helen Wheeler, guided on a successful summit climb by Ed Stuhl, inquired as to the name of the lovely tarn. Ed christened the tiny lake on the spot, and the name has stuck ever since. Actually, the lake is usually under snow, and hence seldom seen except late in exceptionally dry years. During the drought years of 1975-77, and again in 1988, Helen Lake was visible and worthy of its designation.

If you wish to establish a higher base camp than Horse Camp, the bench at Helen Lake is a popular but often crowded site. Except in winter and early spring, runoff water is usually available, and a number of flat, protected campsites have evolved over the years. Increased use of this fragile alpine environment necessitated the initiation of a human waste pack-out policy by the U.S. Forest Service. Better protected, less windy, and less crowded campsites exist at the 9600–9800 foot level below Helen Lake.

Ed Stuhl: A Lifetime with Mt. Shasta

In June 1917, Edward Stuhl walked up the same Sacramento River canyon that John Muir had traveled forty years earlier. When he reached the area in the canyon near Dunsmuir where Muir had first sighted Mt. Shasta, Stuhl was equally overcome. Thus began a life-long association with Mt. Shasta. Stuhl grew up in Austria and spent his summers traveling through the Austrian mountains for his father's stained-glass studio, repairing church windows that had suffered winter storm damage. Years later he recalled that a turning point in his life occurred when he saw the original Wild Bill Hickok and Annie Oakley's "Wild West Show" in Munich, kindling a desire to experience the American West.

Ed and his wife, Rosie, made their way to California and from 1923 to 1946 they worked for William Randolph Hearst at the publisher's famous Wyntoon estate along the McCloud River. During this time Stuhl successfully climbed Mt. Shasta many times. helped with the construction of the cabin at Horse Camp, and indulged his passion of creating beautiful watercolor paintings of Mt. Shasta's wildflowers. For years he was the de-facto custodian of the cabin, and his campfire stories enthralled the many climbers and hikers who met him on the mountain.

Above Helen Lake lies the most strenuous section of the route, a 2500-foot snowfield that steepens to 35-degrees near its top.

Stay right of center of the main drainage, aiming generally toward the right side of the Red Banks, the prominent orange palisades of welded pumice that represent one of Shasta's more recent flows. Constant vigilance is advised as the Red Banks are the source of most of the rockfall in Avalanche Gulch. Allow yourself plenty of time to climb and return before the sun's heat can loosen and dislodge any rocks. Mid-to-late summer is the most dangerous time, although rockfall can occur during any season and at any time. At nearly 12,000 feet, continue climbing to the right of a large rockfield called the Heart. Depending on the time of the year and the previous winter's snowpack, this rock feature can take on a variety of sizes and shapes. The Heart can also be a source of rock-

The Stuhls later settled in a log cabin west of the town of Mount Shasta and lived actively until well into their nineties. They both skied until their eighties, and Ed, who climbed every major mountain in western North America south of Canada, made a solo winter climb of Mexico's 17,887-foot Popocatepetl when he was 76.

Ed's great hope was to see Mt. Shasta preserved as a national or state park, or wilderness area. He died in 1984, at age 97, only a few months before the Mt. Shasta Wilderness Area was designated by the U.S. Congress. Two legacies of Ed live on: a published collection of his exquisite Mt. Shasta wildflower paintings, and the love and appreciation of Mt. Shasta that he instilled in everyone he met.

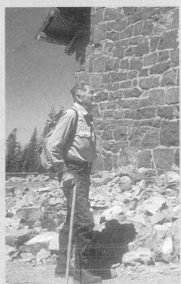

Ed Stuhl

fall. Generally, climbing farther south (climber's right) in this drainage, results in the least exposure to rockfall.

The small saddle between the Red Banks and Thumb Rock at 12,800 feet is a good place to rest, eat and warm up in the sun; a snug alcove can provide protection in case of wind.

There are two main options for the next section: either around or through the Red Banks. The usual way is to walk briefly around and behind the Red Banks on the edge of the Konwakiton Glacier, avoiding the crevasse (called a *bergschrund*, although technically it's a moat here) where the glacier snow has pulled away from the rock. In mid-to-late summer the bergschrund can be quite large, blocking easy return to the Red Banks' crest. Snowbridges across this bergschrund may offer safe passage in the cool of the morning, but be aware that they can be dangerously softened by the afternoon sun.

If your lack of equipment and experience, or your intuition causes doubt about going around the Red Banks, you can backtrack a few hundred feet and climb upward through one of several open gullies in the Red Banks, reaching their top shortly.

Depending upon seasonal conditions, short but steep snow slopes, ice and exposure on this section through or around the Red Banks can be the one area on this route where some climbers might want the comfort of a rope, but unless a partner is skilled in holding falls in the conditions present, a rope can add a false sense of security and the potential to pull off teammates.

Whichever route you choose to ascend the Red Banks, continue climbing along the top of the Red Banks and follow the ridge to its top, a broad snowfield bounded on the north by the Whitney Glacier and on the south by the Konwakiton Glacier.

A short but worthwhile side trip is a brief walk north on the snowfield at the top of the Red Banks. Here, you can enjoy a view of the whole expanse of the Whitney Glacier, the longest glacier in California. In mid-season, Clarence King Lake (within Shastina's crater) and Sisson Lake (on the saddle between Shasta and

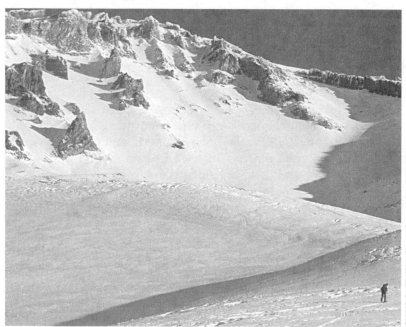

Avalanche Gulch

CHRIS CARR/SHASTA MOUNTAIN GUIDES

Shastina) appear as turquoise jewels against the stark white backdrop of snow.

Continue up "Misery Hill" (either a misnomer or an understatement, depending upon conditions of route and climbers) via the best-quality snow or a faint scree trail to the right of center of the hill. You soon reach the flat summit snowfield. Cross this plateau, heading for an obvious col between the summit pinnacle to the right (E), and a smaller one to the west. The summit snowfield is often wind-and-sun-sculpted into a labyrinth of bizarre and beautiful shapes called "penitentes." During late season, and in years of light snowpack, the twisted cylindrical remains of the old geodetic monument may be seen emerging from snow beneath the southwest face of the summit pinnacle. The bubbling sulfur fumaroles nearby are a reminder that Mt. Shasta is indeed a volcano, active not long ago.

Ascend the summit via easy scrambling on its northwest side, thus concluding Mt. Shasta's most historic and most popular route.

Descend via the same route.

Variation 1a   Left of Heart

Difficulty: 2 (PD)

Time: 1+ days

During unusually dry seasons, and late in the summer, this drainage usually holds snow longer than the traditional route to the right, offering better climbing for those who are experienced on steep slopes. Climb increasingly steep snow fields above Helen Lake until you're beneath the imposing north end of Red Banks.

Depending upon seasonal conditions, several icy chimneys offer challenging passages through these palisades, and in fact ice climbers looking for rare summer practice can often find some near-vertical water ice in some of them. The chimneys become shorter and easier the farther left (N) you go along the Red Banks, although steep snow cornices often overhang at the extreme left end. If so, a steep, short ridge left (N) of the Red Banks abuts the very top of Casaval Ridge, and offers passage around the cornices. You are now atop the Red Banks and at the base of Misery Hill, slightly north of the traditional route, which can be followed to the summit.

Descend the same route, or Route 1.

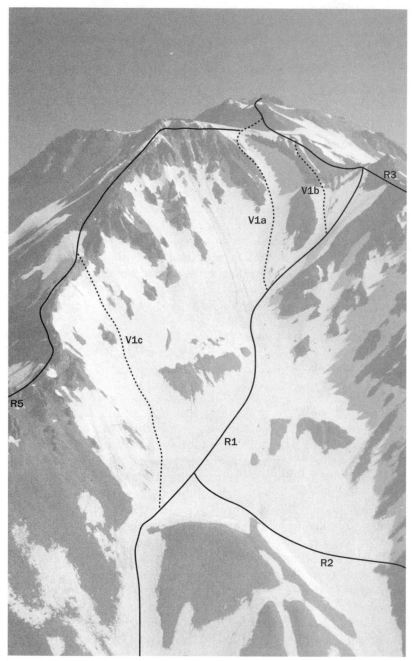

Mt. Shasta from the south-southwest, looking at Avalanche Gulch

Variation 1b   Red Banks Chimneys

DIFFICULTY: 2 (PD)

TIME: 1 day

During times when the Konwakiton Glacier *bergschrund* presents difficulties (see Route 1 description), these variations are enjoyable, time-saving detours. When climbing the traditional route (Route 1), you pass beneath the Red Banks for several hundred feet before reaching a saddle at Thumb Rock. At the lowest point of the Red Banks is a huge, cleft rock outcropping that looks like a caricature valentine. Just right of this "heart" (not the same as the rock island below of that name) is a deep, snow-filled chimney leading all the way to the top of the Red Banks. A few hundred feet right of this chimney is another landmark—an anvil-shaped rock. This rock may also be passed on either side to reach the top of the Red Banks.

Descend via Route 1—although the chimneys may be descended if they are not too icy.

Variation 1c   Upper Casaval Ridge

DIFFICULTY: 2 to 3 (PD+)

TIME: 1+ days

Looking north from Helen Lake, you can see a broad shoulder descending from Casaval Ridge. This shoulder is much less steep than any other rib or gully descending from Casaval Ridge. This is the "second window," a common escape, or bail-out, from Route 5. This route variation is an excellent portal for gaining access to the upper reaches of Casaval Ridge late in the season when the lower parts of the ridge lack snow. Follow Casaval Ridge to its top, then the traditional route (Route 1) to the summit

Descend either your ascent route or Route 1, depending on conditions and time.

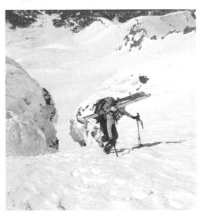

Climbing through the Red Banks

Route 2 OLD SKI BOWL

DIFFICULTY: 1 (F)

ACCESS: Everitt Memorial Highway, Panther Meadows

CAMPSITES: Panther Meadow, old Ski Bowl lodge parking area

TIME: 1 day

The original Ski Bowl was opened in 1959, and it remained in operation until 1978, when weather, financial problems, and a lift-destroying avalanche forced its closure. All that remains is the parking lot. While the Ski Bowl was open, Everitt Memorial Highway was regularly plowed its full 14-mile length. This enabled year-round access to Sargents Ridge and many excellent cross-country and ski-mountaineering routes. Now the road is plowed only as far as Bunny Flat, and the remaining 3 miles to Panther Meadows and the Ski Bowl are left to thaw on their own, usually by the end of June.

From the Ski Bowl parking lot, a maze of old dirt service roads winds upward through a cirque to the location of the old top terminal at 9200 feet, where several radiotelephone antennas remain. From this location, head directly north until intersecting Green Butte Ridge, the southern margin of vast Avalanche Gulch. Follow the ridge to a gap just north of Point 9572, then contour left to the traditional route (Route 1) near Helen Lake. Since the last 3 miles of Everitt Memorial Highway are no longer plowed, access to this route is seldom open until late June or early July. By then, there are long stretches of exposed scree and talus on the climbing route. Descend your route of ascent.

Variation 2 Green Butte Ridge to Sargents Ridge (R 3)

DIFFICULTY: 2 (PD)

TIME: 1+ days

Instead of traversing left to the traditional John Muir route, continue climbing Green Butte Ridge until it joins Sargents Ridge at 12,000 feet. Follow Sargents Ridge (R 3) to its juncture with the traditional route (R 1) at Thumb Rock. Descend via the climbing route.

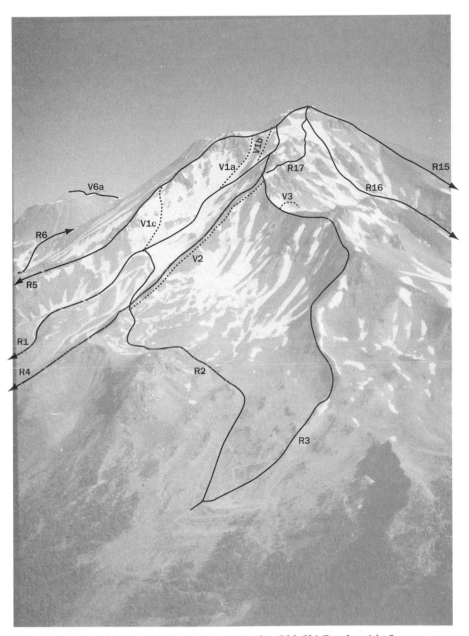

Mt. Shasta from the south, looking at the Old Ski Bowl, with Sargents Ridge on the left, and the Clear Creek route on the right

Route 3 SARGENTS RIDGE

DIFFICULTY: 2 (PD)
ACCESS: Everitt Memorial Highway
CAMPSITES: Panther Meadow, old Ski Bowl
lodge parking area
TIME: 1+ days

Named for John Sargent, a forest ranger who enjoyed climbing Mt. Shasta in the 1940s, this ridge is an excellent winter route because of its general lack of avalanche exposure. Summer popularity has waned in recent years because late openings of the last 3 miles of Everitt Memorial Highway have prevented easy access. By mid-to-late summer, lack of snow on the route makes for some unpleasant climbing over talus and scree. In winter and spring, however, it's worth the effort to ski or snowshoe from Bunny Flat to a base camp in the old Ski Bowl to climb this route.

From any of many good campsites in the Ski Bowl cirque, climb northeast on gentle shoulders that join the ridge proper. A good landmark on the crest above is Shastarama Point (Point 11,135), a major, turreted crag. Beyond this large outcropping, the ridge flattens for a quarter mile. Here you'll have excellent views of the Mud Creek and the Konwakiton glaciers, as well as the impressive, precipitous depths of Mud Creek Canyon. Continue upward on

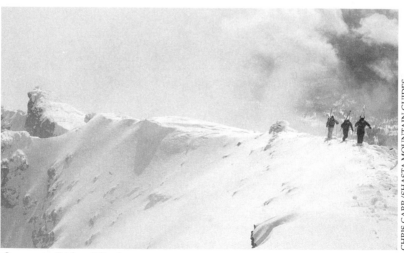

Sargents Ridge Climb

CHRIS CARR/SHASTA MOUNTAIN GUIDES

the steepening ridge, avoiding obstacles and exposure by bearing left. Join Route 1 at the Red Banks-Thumb Rock saddle and follow it to the summit.

Descend the climbing route or Route 1 to the Ski Bowl traverse (R 2).

Variation 3 Traverse to Mud Creek Glacier

DIFFICULTY: 2 (PD)

TIME: 1 day

From the long, flat ridge just beyond Shastarama Point, a short traverse to the east takes you to the small Mud Creek Glacier. This glacier has a stark, alpine beauty but is seldom visited. There is also a beautiful hidden lake behind Shastarama Point.

Descend via the approach route.

Route 4 GREEN BUTTE RIDGE

DIFFICULTY: 1 to 2 (PD-)

ACCESS: Everitt Memorial Highway

CAMPSITE: Bunny Flat

TIME: 1+ days

This route and the Old Ski Bowl route (R 2) share a distinction: while not particularly aesthetic or notable, these routes are popular among climbers with limited time because one can start climbing right from a parking lot and avoid any hike into a base camp. In recent years, however, with road plowing to the Ski Bowl discontinued, Green Butte Ridge has become more popular as an accessible and safe winter route.

From the parking area at Bunny Flat, climb northeast on gentle, forested slopes until you're above timberline and level with Green Butte, the large, rounded shoulder at 9200 feet which juts outward to the south. Continue northeast on Green Butte ridge to join the Sargents Ridge route (R 3), or traverse to the traditional route (R 1) as in the Ski Bowl (R 2) route description.

Descend via the climbing route.

Route 5   CASAVAL RIDGE

DIFFICULTY: 2 to 3 (PD+)

ACCESS: Everitt Memorial Highway

CAMPSITES: Horse Camp, Helen Lake, Sand Flat, Bunny Flat

TIME: 2 to 2+ days

Casaval Ridge is the striking, cockscomb-like ridge north of Avalanche Gulch. Worldly mountaineers compare it to famous classics of the Alps. The route offers an excellent winter ascent and an airy, stimulating spring and early-summer climb. Ample bivvy sites add to the attraction of the climb. After early summer the route is not recommended due to lack of snow and much loose rock.

From the Sierra Club Foundation cabin at Horse Camp, a broad toe of the ridge is only a few hundred yards north. Climb this wide ridge to about 9800 feet, where it makes a jog to the left at an excellent bivvy site and joins serrated Casaval Ridge proper. The first

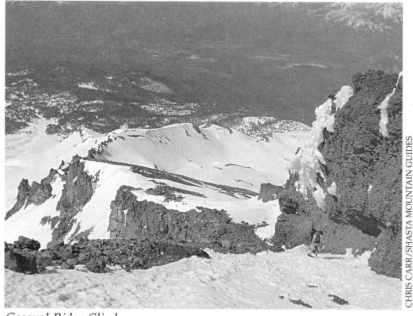

Casaval Ridge Climb

part of the ridge is fairly low-angle; you can go around towers blocking the way on either side, but left (N) is usually easier. The ridge begins to increase in steepness at 10,800 feet, a little above Helen Lake, which is visible to the right (S). This part of the ridge, called the "first window," offers escape to Helen Lake via moderate slopes on the right. The route steepens at this point, but there are many wide sections.

A second escape, the "second window," occurs at 11,800. Here, another broad, moderate slope curves down into Avalanche Gulch above Helen Lake. (During times of avalanche danger, it's unwise to descend into main Avalanche Gulch.) There are a few short, steep sections on the ridge at 13,000 feet. This route joins Route 1 at 13,500 feet and continues to the summit.

Descend either the climbing route or one of the Avalanche Gulch routes as time and conditions dictate.

Variation 5   The West Face Gully

DIFFICULTY:	2 (PD)
ACCESS:	Everitt Memorial Highway
CAMPSITES:	Horse Camp, Sand Flat, Bunny Flat
TIME:	1 to 2 days

North of Casaval Ridge is a beautiful, long gully that begins in Hidden Valley at 9700 feet and ends nearly 4000 feet later at the broad snowfield at the base of Misery Hill. This rarely done route retains snow long into summer, and is an excellent alternative route when Casaval Ridge is too rocky and devoid of snow to be pleasant or safe.

It is best to begin the climb from a high camp in Hidden Valley. From the Sierra Club Foundation cabin at Horse Camp, traverse and gradually climb north. Cross several gullies until you reach Hidden Valley at 9200 feet. A good landmark to aim for from the cabin is a spire of rock (Point 9487) that coincides closely with true north. Once you reach the ridge below and west of the spire, you can descend easily into Hidden Valley, an extensive flat basin that makes an excellent, well-protected high camp.

If you choose to begin the climb from the lower stretches of Casaval Ridge, you must traverse north to the gully. When the gully begins to narrow at its top, stay left of the dark orange palisades—the westernmost volcanic flow of the Red Banks.

Descend either the route of ascent or Cascade Gulch and the West Ridge (R6).

Route 6 **CASCADE GULCH**

DIFFICULTY: 1 to 2 (PD-)
ACCESS: Everitt Memorial Highway
CAMPSITES: Bunny Flat, Sand Flat, Horse Camp, Hidden Valley
TIME: 1 to 2 days

The famous geologist Clarence King, who is credited with discovering the glaciers on Mt. Shasta, the first glaciers to be identified in the United States, made one of the first ascents of this route, in 1870. Clarence King Lake, within Shastina's crater, was named after him.

From the Sierra Club Foundation cabin at Horse Camp, traverse and gradually climb north. Cross several gullies until you reach Hidden Valley at 9200 feet. A good landmark to aim for from the cabin is a spire of rock (Point 9487) that coincides closely with true north. Once you reach the ridge below and west of the spire, you can descend easily into Hidden Valley, an extensive flat basin that makes an excellent, well-protected high camp. From there, stay left of the main watercourse—and the waterfall at the head of Hidden Valley—and climb upward to the 12,000-foot saddle between Shasta and Shastina.

Climb east along Shasta's wide west ridge, avoiding some steep drop-offs onto the Whitney Glacier. As the ridge narrows, follow the narrow snowfield above the Whitney Glacier bergschrund to a point atop the Red Banks and a little west of Misery Hill. Be prepared for short sections of roped climbing if it's necessary to cross the bergschrund. You can avoid glacier travel by following the serrated upper ridge west of the Whitney Glacier; careful route finding, generally climbing toward the southwest, is necessary to avoid some short, steep sections. Join Route 1 and continue to the summit.

Descend the climbing route or Route 1.

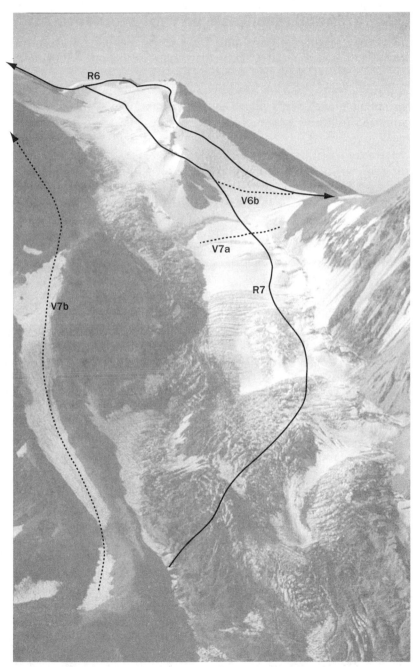

The Whitney Glacier

Variation 6a Ascent of Shastina

DIFFICULTY: 1 (F)

TIME: 1 day

From the Shasta–Shastina saddle a short scramble leads west to Shastina's summit pinnacle. Shastina's crater is over a half mile across and several hundred feet deep. Clarence King Lake looks like a turquoise jewel when it becomes free of snow in midsummer.

Variation 6b Upper Whitney Glacier to Summit

DIFFICULTY: 2 to 3 (AD+)

TIME: 2 days

The upper Whitney Glacier is very smooth compared to the chaotic middle and lower parts of the glacier, and offers pleasant climbing without many crevasses. From the Shasta-Shastina saddle, ascend the west ridge a few hundred feet until the easiest entry to the glacier presents itself. Usually several snowfields spill over onto the glacier from the ridge, providing convenient access. Avoid descending directly from the saddle to the glacier, as a *bergschrund* and icy cliffs can be dangerous.

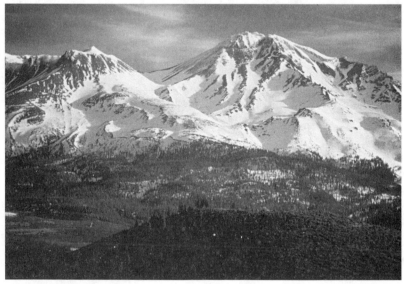

Shastina and Shasta

If you climb too high on the west ridge, some short rock faces prevent easy entry to the glacier. Climb upward, curving east on the glacier, and follow rock ribs to the summit plateau. Descend either the climbing route or the west ridge (R6).

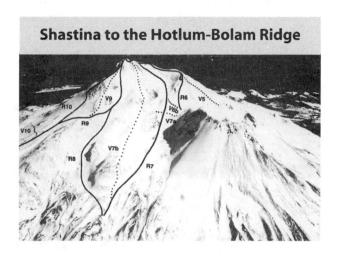

Shastina to the Hotlum-Bolam Ridge

From Diller Canyon clockwise around Shastina to the Whitney Glacier are many shallow gullies. The climbing is generally arduous because of large amounts of talus and loose rock. Diller Canyon is often climbed in conjunction with a ski descent, but in times of little snow, loose 4th class rock makes the last 1000 feet undesirable.

Route 7 WHITNEY GLACIER

DIFFICULTY: 2 to 3 (AD+)

ACCESS: Whitney Falls, North Gate, or Bolam Trailheads. An eastern fork of the Bolam road allows higher access for 4WD vehicles.

CAMPSITES: Whitney, Bolam and unnamed intermittent creeks

TIME: 2+ days

The Summit Monument

In 1875 the U.S. Coast and Geodetic Survey decided it was necessary to increase the accuracy of their maps. Signal towers were
planned for Mt. Shasta, Mt. Saint Helena (near Clear Lake, California),
and Mt. Lola (west of Reno, Nevada) to be included as part of the survey grid. On April 30, 1875, John Muir and local guide Jerome Fay
climbed Shasta to take barometric measurements and study the fea-
sibility of placing a tower on the summit. A fierce storm caught the
pair on the summit and, unable to descend, they spent the night
huddled over the summit's hot sulfur fumaroles. Muir's account of
the experience, "A Snow Storm on Mt. Shasta," is one of his most
famous writings.

The signal tower, with polished copper top, was fabricated in San
Francisco and carried in pieces to the summit, where it was assem-
bled and anchored in place. In August of 1878, Coast and Geodetic
Survey assistant Benjamin Colonna spent nine continuous days on
Shasta's summit waiting for favorable conditions. Finally, on August
1, Colonna exchanged flashes with surveyors on the other two
peaks. The line from Mt. Shasta to Mt. Saint Helena, 192 miles, was the
longest terrestrial distance ever measured, surpassing the previous
record of 169 miles from Spain across the Mediterranean to Algeria.

The Whitney Glacier was named for Professor Josiah D. Whitney,
the leader of the California Geologic Survey and of the scientific
exploration of Mt. Shasta in 1862. This is California's largest glacier.
The glacier stretches for well over 2 miles, and its foot is covered
with an enormous quantity of rubble and debris.

A base camp on the lower glacier is an experience for the sens-
es: With the towering flanks of Shastina rising over 4000 feet to the
west and the long, broad Whitney-Bolam ridge bordering the cav-
ernous canyon on the east, the tableau looks like the Alaska Range
or the Himalaya. In early evening's shadows or by moonlight, the
scale and the vastness of the scene seem totally different from their
daytime aspects. Add to this the constant creaking and grinding of
the glacial ice, the irregular sounds of water, and the cannonades
and crescendos of rockfalls and breaking seracs, all contributing to
a dramatic alpine setting.

After the survey work was completed, the monument was abandoned for any further scientific use. In fact, it became adorned with graffiti as climbers scratched and painted their names on the tower.

In 1903, guide Tom Watson led Alice Cousins astride horse "Old Jump Up" to the summit via the Clear Creek route. It was the first horse to reach Shasta's pinnacle, and the picture of them next to the monument was used in "Ripley's Believe It Or Not" features for many years. Then, in the winter of 1903, the monument collapsed, a victim of Shasta's severe winds and weather. The crushed cylinder can still be seen at the west base of the summit pinnacle. The copper reflector was brought down in 1949 and is on display at the Sisson Museum in the town of Mount Shasta.

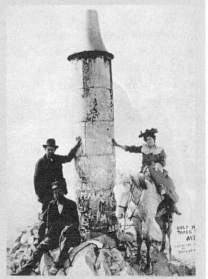

PHOTO COURTESY OF ED STUHL COLLECTION

Guide Tom Watson with Alice Cousins astride "Old Jump Up" at the summit

From either the Whitney Creek, North Gate, or the Bolam road access, there are many base-camp choices. In winter or early spring, you can approach easily on skis, with several comfortable benches for base camp. In summer, it's usually best to set up base camp on the flat lower glacier. There are also some miniature meadows and springs near timberline just west of the glacier terminus, but these can be difficult to find.

Climbing the lower glacier is relatively straightforward, but there might be minor route-finding problems in late summer and fall as small crevasses begin to open. Avoid venturing close to Shastina's flanks because of the threat of rockfall, and be wary of a similar threat from the upper slopes of Shasta. The center of the lower glacier is generally safest.

When snow still covers most of the glacier, the big icefall adjacent to the Shasta–Shastina saddle is the only major obstacle along the route. In early season several paths may become visible, but the glacial geography is an ever-changing kaleidoscope in three dimensions, and you must be prepared to use your best skills and judgment to improvise a route. In late summer and fall, the enormity of the crevasses and of the *bergschrund* spanning the glacier's full width, and the precariousness of the seracs, give an entirely different and very serious condition to the icefall. By then, literally acres of seracs have toppled and avalanched, mostly during the heat of midday. Either side of this icefall section can offer reasonably safe passage. The east side is a little more direct; the west side offers the sanctuary of the Shasta-Shastina saddle, but can be steeper in places. Above the icefall, follow the smooth upper glacier to the summit plateau.

Descend the climbing route.

Variation 7a   Whitney Icefall for Serac and Ice Climbing

DIFFICULTY: 3 (AD)
TIME: 2+ days

When the ice conditions are at their best, the main icefall is a worthy objective for ice-climbing practice. There is sufficient ice most of the time except in midwinter, when the icefall is covered with snow. In summer, warm temperatures can create extremely unstable conditions within the icefall, and seracs can topple at any time.

Variation 7b   Whitney-Bolam Ridge

DIFFICULTY: 1 to 2 (PD-)
TIME: 1 to 2 days

This seldom-done variation is very nice when there is sufficient snowpack; without the snowpack, it's an unenjoyable trudge through loose talus. This ridge can provide a quicker descent to base camp than the Whitney Glacier itself, and in times of adequate snow it is an outstanding ski descent route. The route may be done in its entirety, or you can traverse east from the Whitney Glacier onto the ridge to avoid the Whitney icefall.

From base camp the route appears as a series of gentle shoulders arranged like ascending steps. Follow the path of least resistance over the steps; bearing southwest is usually easiest. At about

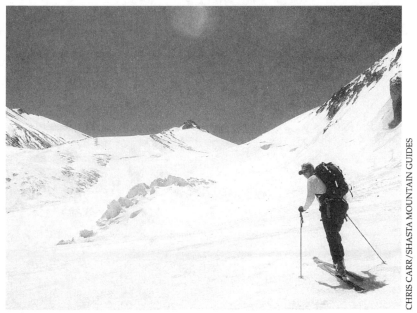

Whitney Glacier ski tour

12,000 feet, the steps give way to a continuous slope which can be followed to the summit plateau.

Descend the ascent route.

Route 8   WEST BOLAM GLACIER

DIFFICULTY: 2 (PD-)

ACCESS: Whitney, North Gate, or Bolam road

CAMPSITES: Bolam Creek and numerous morainal steps and benches

TIME: 1 to 2 days

The Bolam Glacier is very broad and smooth—easy to climb for a glacier its size. It is an excellent glacier for newcomers to glacier climbing, or as a first glacier climb on Mt. Shasta. The routes are general, and several variations are possible. You can also escape, if necessary, to the wide ridge to the west at several points. Major difficulties on the upper glacier are a long obvious *bergschrund* and some small crevasses. Although this route is not the easiest way to the glacier, the balance may be tipped in its favor if residual snow

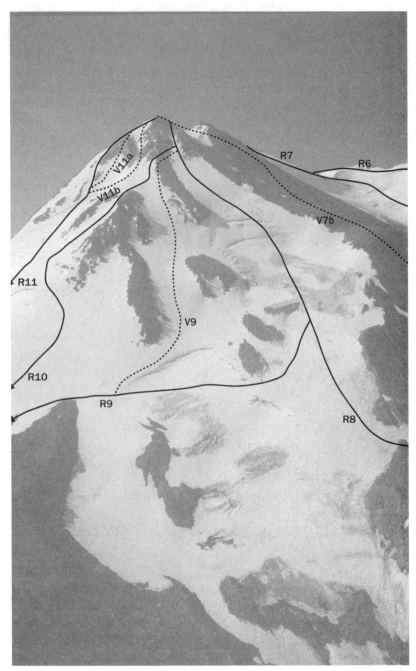

Mt. Shasta from the north-northwest, showing the Bolam Glacier

or other conditions render the northeast approach longer or more difficult. For some, the rugged beauty of the glacier terminus is its own reward.

The Whitney Glacier base camps can position you for the climb, but it's more advantageous to traverse higher under the Bolam Glacier to a campsite on one of the many morainal shelves. Climb the broad west side of the glacier, passing two very large rock islands on their right sides. From steeper slopes on the glacier's upper reaches, you can attain the summit plateau via mixed climbing to the west, or good, short gullies to the east.

Descend the climbing route.

Route 9 EAST BOLAM GLACIER

DIFFICULTY: 2 (PD-)

ACCESS: North Gate Trailhead

CAMPSITES: North Gate, surrounding forest. The many flat and sandy lateral moraines between the Hotlum and Bolam glaciers also offer excellent campsites and numerous sources of water.

TIME: 1 to 2 days

When the North Gate road is open, often by mid-to-late June, this is the best access to the Bolam Glacier. The approach hike or ski is easy, and any of the base camps are comfortable. Choose one of the many excellent high camps described in Route 10 and traverse to the glacier from the vicinity of 10,000 feet. You can also continue west from North Gate, past very large, descending benches to the jumbled moraines at the glacier's foot. Climb to the west of the two large rock islands, and from there follow Route 8 to the summit.

Descend the climbing route.

Variation 9 Bolam Gully

DIFFICULTY: 3 (AD)

TIME: 1 to 2 days

Climb the long, shallow gully left (E) of the two large rock islands described in the two previous routes. The snow in this gully is usually in excellent condition, although it can sometimes be icy. When

The Mt. Shasta Book

level with the top of the second rock island, you can bear right and follow steep mixed climbing to the summit area, or else traverse east to Route 10 and follow that route to the summit.

Descend either the climbing route or Route 10, depending on conditions and time.

Route 10 **HOTLUM-BOLAM RIDGE**

DIFFICULTY: 2 (PD)

ACCESS: North Gate Trailhead

CAMPSITES: North Gate, surrounding forest. The many flat and sandy lateral moraines between the Hotlum and Bolam glaciers also offer excellent campsites and numerous sources of water.

TIME: 1 to 2 days

The Hotlum-Bolam ridge route is truly a route for all seasons. The access road takes you to an unexpectedly high elevation. The trail through North Gate and the surrounding forest is pleasant, and campsites are numerous with water close at hand. During winter, when parts of the mountain's north side experience a weather "rainshadow" effect, road access reaches high enough to enable a fairly direct and gentle ski or snowshoe ascent to a suitable base camp. The most difficult season for this route is often late summer and fall, when it often becomes quite icy. In general, the ridge is not prone to avalanche danger.

Ascend the trail through the North Gate area, the shallow ravine between a large mesa-like lava flow on the left (E), and large, rugged outcroppings on the right (W). Several base camp choices are possible. In early summer, when there is still sufficient snow on the north slopes of the mesa, it can be easily ascended. The top of this formation is a descending series of broad, sandy benches protected from weather and usually offering season-long water in shallow gullies from many accumulated snow drifts. These benches provide some of the most comfortable above-timberline camping anywhere on Shasta.

During late summer, when the mesa's north slopes are devoid of snow, loose talus and scree make a direct ascent to the mesa's top very unpleasant. In that season, continue around the mesa's

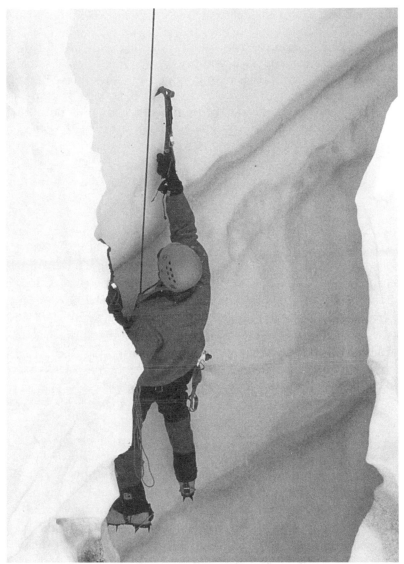

Ice climbing practice on a crevasse wall, Hotlum Glacier

west shoulder, gain elevation, and cut back to the left (E) on wide talus ramps to a point midway on the series of benches atop the formation. You can also camp a short distance west of the mesa near an unnamed all-season stream, or continue up past a lovely, small waterfall to excellent campsites between 9000 and 10,000 feet.

The climbing route follows broad snow slopes toward the obvious Hotlum-Bolam ridge. If you bear right, you'll find it's steep, but you'll gain the ridge quickly. In good snow conditions, it's better to contour left, skirt the bergschrund and crevasse hazards on the Hotlum's west lobe, and then follow a broad snow ramp that angles up and to the right to a large, flat platform at 12,800 feet on

The Exploration and Naming of Shasta's Glaciers

Shortly after the 1849 California gold rush, Governor John Downey appointed Josiah Whitney as State Geologist, bestowing the task of completing a geologic survey with special attention to mineral resources. Whitney's assistant was William Brewer. In 1862 they followed the Sacramento River north to Mt. Shasta, climbing the peak on September 12, and obtaining barometric readings at the summit to compute an elevation of 14,440 feet. This was then considered the highest point in the United States.

After the climb, Brewer wrote a letter to an old friend, George Jarvis Brush, Professor of Metallurgy at Yale University, describing his adventures on Shasta. One of Brush's students, Clarence King, happened by the office and read Brewer's letter. For King, who eventually rose to the directorship of the U.S. Geological Survey, this was a pivotal moment. He immediately volunteered as an assistant field geologist to Whitney's California survey.

While doing field work on Shasta's slopes in 1864, King and Brewer discovered an unusual milky-looking stream, similar to the silty runoff from a glacier. King inquired, and Brewer replied that he had climbed the peak without discovering any glaciers. Evidence of an ancient glacial epoch in North America had already been recognized, and climbers had been on Cascade glaciers farther north, but American geologists and glaciologists all believed that no active glaciers remained anywhere in the United States.

King returned to Mt. Shasta in the fall of 1870 as director of the government-sponsored Geologic Survey of the Fortieth Parallel. When King and his assistants climbed Mt. Shasta in September, 1870, the ridge. If the lower ridge and the broad ramp are icy, you can traverse left on snowfields that skirt the west side of the middle Hotlum Glacier, then curve around and up to the platform at 12,800 feet. Be prepared for roped glacier travel if you plan to venture onto the Hotlum Glacier. From the platform, the imposing Hotlum headwall looms to the left in full view.

Follow a triangular snowfield leading up the ridge to the west toward two obvious rock towers, or "ears," which can be seen from

they ascended via the huge saddle between Shasta and Shastina, and were rewarded with their first views of an active glacier in the United States. Shasta's great northside "ice river" was later named for King's mentor, Josiah Whitney. King later told Brewer, "That stream haunted me for years, until I got on Mt. Shasta and found the glaciers." The discovery was considered one of the most important geologic events of the decade.

The credit for naming Shasta's other glaciers belongs to the famous Western explorer Major John Wesley Powell. Powell was a brilliant scholar who collected over two dozen dictionaries of Native American languages and dialects. During 1879 he came to northern California to study the Wintun tribe, and climbed Mt. Shasta on November 1, 1879. Afterward, he named Shasta's four other major glaciers with Wintun words in honor of the tribe: Hotlum ("steep"), Bolam ("big" or "great"), Konwakiton ("muddy"), and Wintun (the tribal name). The names were inscribed in official records maintained by the US Geographic Board in 1897.

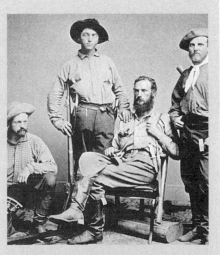

California Geological Survey of 1864. William Brewer is seated; Clarence King is standing at the right.

well down the mountain and which are good points of reference. Pass these towers on the right and climb through large broken blocks on the ridge. Follow the ridge to the summit. If wind or ice makes the uppermost ridge undesirable, you can continue past the two ears on their right, pass through any of several notches on the ridge, and ascend an easy snow gully hidden on the ridge's west side. This gully can be followed until several short, shallow ribs offer easy return to the ridge just short of the summit. You can also continue climbing in the gully to the hot springs beneath the summit pinnacle. In late summer and fall, large sections of this route can become icy.

Descend the climbing route.

Variation 10a Side trip to the Chicago Glacier from the North

DIFFICULTY: 1 to 2 (F-PD)

TIME: 1 day

From base camp atop the mesa, ascend west a few hundred vertical feet and traverse southeast to this seldom-visited and isolated glacier.

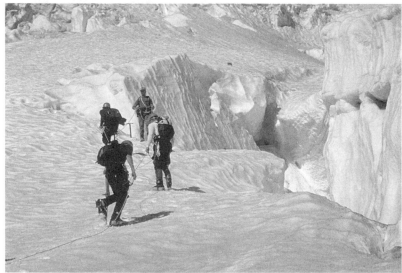

Glacier travel practice on Hotlum Glacier

North and Northeast Sides, Hotlum and Wintun Glaciers

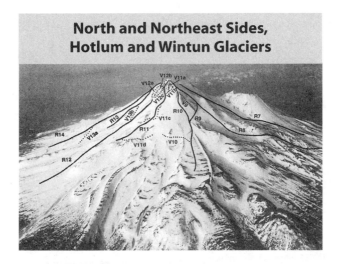

ROUTE 11   HOTLUM GLACIER

DIFFICULTY: 3 (AD)

ACCESS: Brewer Creek Trailhead

CAMPSITES: Brewer Creek, Gravel Creek, moraine lakes and meadows

TIME: 2 days

From an impressive rock headwall beginning at nearly 13,000 feet, the Hotlum Glacier descends in a gentle S-turn past 3 spectacular icefalls. At the lowest icefall—a huge broken and convoluted formation just right (N) of a prominent rock prow—the glacier levels out and ends in several acres of fascinating ice ribs. Spread out below this terminus are rugged morainal hummocks and small, hidden lakes. Finally, the headwaters of Gravel Creek and other smaller streams emerge into the red-fir and hemlock forests below.

Several fine base camp areas are found in the Brewer and Gravel Creek drainages, from which the glacier may be climbed to one of the summit variations. You can also establish a high camp on a prominent rock prow at 11,700 feet below and north of the middle icefall. In spring and early summer the glacier is predominantly smooth from accumulated snow. In late summer and fall, the curved path of the Hotlum Glacier becomes a maze of crevasses, and careful route finding is necessary. At this time the icefalls also come into their best condition for serac climbing.

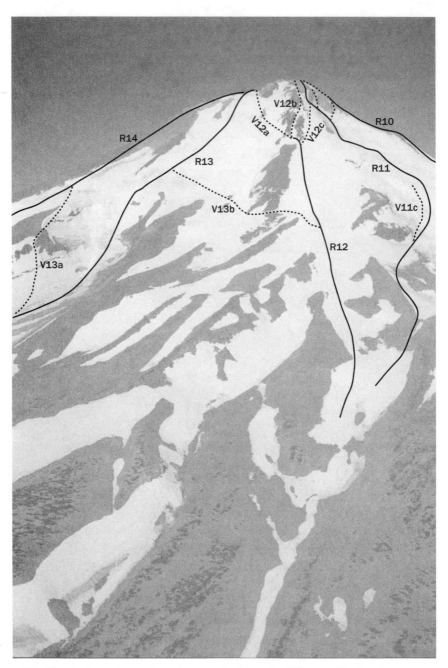

Mt. Shasta from the east-northeast, showing the Wintun Glacier

The climbing route ascends to the right (N) of the lower icefall, then gradually curves upward and left (S) of the middle icefall. Continue upward, again gradually bearing right (N), until reaching the broad upper glacier, which is slightly below and to the left of the upper icefall. At this point, although the slope remains moderate, several crevasses may extend completely across the glacier. In late summer and in times of diminished snow, these abysses can halt easy upward progress. The ridge to the left (S), which becomes most evident above the lower icefall, offers an escape at several points. You can then follow this ridge to the summit.

The usual challenging finish is to climb the steep, often icy couloirs just left of the headwall to an area atop the headwall, and just northeast of the summit pinnacle. From most points on the middle and upper reaches of the Hotlum Glacier, you can also traverse right (N) to join Route 10, the Hotlum-Bolam ridge route.

Descend the climbing route or Route 10.

Variation 11a   Hotlum Glacier Headwall

DIFFICULTY: 3+ (D-)

TIME: 2 days

From the *bergschrund* climb increasingly steep snow to the very apex of the glacier beneath the rock headwall. Three to five rock pitches (some class 5.8), depending upon route finding, lead to easier climbing just below the summit pinnacle. The combination of exposure, some loose rock, required commitment, and high altitude make this one of the most difficult routes on the mountain.

Variation 11b   Hotlum Headwall Ice Gully

DIFFICULTY: 3+ (D-) mixed climbing (rock and ice) up to very difficult

TIME: 2 days

Just right (N) of the obvious headwall in Variation 11a is one of Shasta's longest, steepest ice gullies. In the fall, hard water-ice abounds and this gully is one of the best ice climbs on Mt. Shasta. In summer, scattered snow patches can thinly cover parts of the ice to create deceptively safe but actually very dangerous conditions. The route is easy to follow but is steep, and ends at easier climbing below the summit pinnacle.

Variation 11c
Hotlum Icefalls

DIFFICULTY: 3 (AD)

TIME: 2 days

The three Hotlum icefalls offer Shasta's best and most accessible serac climbing. A careful choice of your base camp or high camp will enable you to enjoy excellent ice climbing only minutes from your tent. The lower icefall, situated at the front of the huge Hotlum amphitheater, conveys a feeling of grandeur, and its mazes of seracs are exciting to explore. In addition, the broad and gentle terminus below the lower icefall is

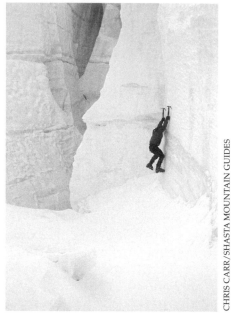

Serac bouldering on Hotlum Glacier

CHRIS CARR/SHASTA MOUNTAIN GUIDES

excellent for beginning glacier and ice training. Plan your high-camp location and climbing activities carefully, because seracs on the middle and lower icefalls may weaken and collapse during warm weather.

Variation 11d   Side Trip to the Chicago Glacier from the South

DIFFICULTY: 1 to 2 (F-PD)

TIME: 1 day

From any of the base camps for the preceding Hotlum Glacier climbing routes, you can traverse north about 0.5 mile with little gain or loss in elevation to the Chicago Glacier. Seldom visited, this glacier has received long-term scientific attention and study by the University of Chicago Geology Department because of its apparent growth. You can also reach the glacier by a gentle traverse over talus from where the whitebark-pine flats meet the undulating morainal hills in the vicinity of Gravel Creek.

Route 12 HOTLUM-WINTUN RIDGE

DIFFICULTY: 2 (PD)

ACCESS: Brewer Creek Trailhead

CAMPSITES: Brewer Creek, Gravel Creek, moraine lakes and meadows

TIME: 1+ days

This fine route is one of the most scenic on Shasta's east side, and an excellent alternative to the often-crowded Avalanche Gulch climbs. The first ascent was likely made by the ubiquitous Norman Clyde in September 1935. If the route is followed correctly, almost no glacier technicalities will be encountered. The name "ridge" is a slight misnomer as most of the route follows broad, permanent snowfields located between the Hotlum and the Wintun glaciers. Above 12,400 feet, the ridge separating the glaciers becomes very distinct, and it is one of the variations to the summit.

The Brewer Creek meadows at timberline make an excellent base camp and offer a very direct start to the climb. Follow the snowfield in the main drainage upward, climbing left (S) of the lower Hotlum icefall and rock cliffs, where incipient crevasses could be troublesome. Continue upward to 12,400 feet, where the ridge becomes distinct. From this high point, choose one of the following summit variations.

Variation 12a Traverse Left (South)

DIFFICULTY: 2 (PD)

TIME: 1+ days

Traverse left (S) to the upper snowfields at the right (N) side of the Wintun Glacier. Pass a solitary, triangular rock island, then climb back to the right and upward to the rock palisades descending from the summit area. Follow the cliff line to the left (W) until encountering the summit snowfield. Curve around to the north to ascend the summit pinnacle. When there is abundant, stable snow on the route this variation is safe, direct and enjoyable. If there is ice, bad visibility, or concern about nearby crevasses, consider the next variation.

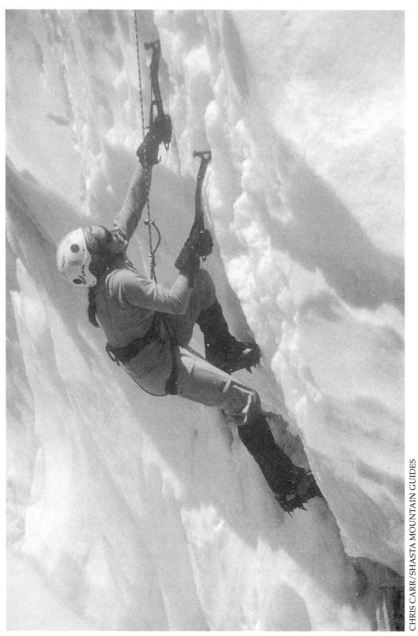

Ice climbing on the Hotlum Glacier

Variation 12b   Rock Ridge Direct

DIFFICULTY: 2 (PD+)

TIME: 1+ days

Climb directly up the Hotlum-Wintun rock ridge that begins at 12,400 feet. With careful route finding, the ridge is 3rd class. If 4th class sections are encountered, they are usually very short, and avoidable by traversing to easier climbing. In ice, verglas, or bad weather, a rope would be advisable. The ridge ends almost directly at the summit.

Variation 12c   Traverse Right (North)

DIFFICULTY: 2 to 3 (PD+)

TIME: 1+ days

This third alternative angles right (N) at the ridge break at 12,400 feet and follows a steep snowfield which skirts the left side of the Hotlum headwall. As this snowfield-cum-gully narrows, stay left of a thin rock rib and climb to easy ground at the summit area.

DESCENDING THE EASTSIDE ROUTES

An eastside descent is potentially hazardous, and forethought should be given to all the variables. Generally, what you have just climbed is fresh and familiar in your mind, and for this reason should be the descent of choice.

If key features and landmarks are noted on the ascent, they can be very useful during the descent. If snow conditions change, visibility or weather worsens, or darkness falls, the two snow variations (Variation 12a and Variation 12c) become very dangerous with unexpected dropoffs and/or crevasses not far from the safe route. Wands or flagging should be placed at critical points on the ascent to mark the route. The rock ridge (Variation 12b), although slower going than the snow variations, avoids any serious dropoffs. At 12,400 feet, continue the descent on the broad snowfield.

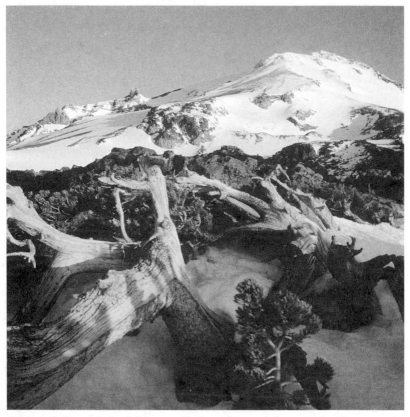

Krummholz whitebark pines and the eastern slopes of Mt. Shasta, near the Clear Creek climbing route

---

Route 13 **WINTUN GLACIER**

DIFFICULTY: 2 to 3 (PD+)

ACCESS: Brewer Creek Trailhead

CAMPSITES: Brewer Creek, Gravel Creek, moraine lakes and meadows

TIME: 1+ days

The Wintun Glacier, named for a local Indian tribe, has many different sections. The upper glacier is wide and clean, and from a beginning just below the east face of the summit pinnacle, the east

108

tongue of the glacier descends smoothly to plateaus between Brewer and Ash creeks. The southeast tongue of the glacier pours over a precipitous icefall and into steep Ash Creek canyon. The lower glacier is an interesting maze of crisscrossing crevasses, and the icefall offers fine practice climbing.

You can establish a base camp near Brewer Creek, or one closer to the glacier by traversing south to the highest of three flat hills seen silhouetted on the ridge south of Brewer Creek. From these hills, you can see most of the route, and a descending traverse will take you to the lower glacier. Except for spring and early summer, some talus will be encountered on this traverse—try to scout ahead to avoid the loosest sections. Pass the icefall on either side, depending on snow conditions, and on where the least debris from above appears to be falling. Easier climbing on the left side of the glacier leads to the summit snowfield.

Descend the climbing route or Wintun Ridge (R 14).

Variation 13a   Traverse to Wintun Ridge

DIFFICULTY: 2 (PD-)

TIME: 1+ days

If conditions on the lower Wintun Glacier and the icefall appear unstable, or debris is raining down from above, you can traverse south out of the canyon to Wintun Ridge. Climb upward on the broad ridge to the summit snowfield, or traverse to the upper Wintun Glacier and follow it to the summit.

Descend the climbing route.

Variation 13b   Brewer Creek Approach
to the Wintun Glacier

DIFFICULTY: 2 (PD-)

TIME: 1+ days

Using this approach you can avoid the lower Wintun Glacier and its icefall entirely, while gaining the easier middle and upper reaches of the glacier. From the Brewer Creek drainage, follow snowfields upward and to the south. Attain the broad, eastern tongue of the Wintun Glacier and follow it to the upper glacier and the summit snowfield.

Route 14   WINTUN RIDGE

DIFFICULTY: 1 to 2 (F)

ACCESS: Clear Creek Trailhead or Brewer Creek (longer)

CAMPSITES: Clear Creek, Pilgrim Creek's many intermittent meadows and springs

TIME: 1 day

This ridge is relatively easy, has excellent views, and, during the right conditions, offers a superb ski descent as fine as any on Mt. Shasta. From a base camp above Clear Creek, Cold Creek, or Pilgrim Creek, climb the wide, lower ridge by the best snowfields. The middle and upper sections of the route are generally clean and smooth, but avoid dropoffs to either side of the ridge, as well as a small, south tongue of the Wintun Glacier. Attain the summit snowfield at its southeast end and follow it to the summit pinnacle.

Descend the climbing route.

Variation 14   Side Trip to Watkins Glacier

DIFFICULTY: 1 to 2

TIME: 1 day

From the 11,000 feet area on Wintun Ridge, a short southward traverse brings you to the Watkins Glacier. This small glacier and cirque are beautiful, and the detour is well worth the time.

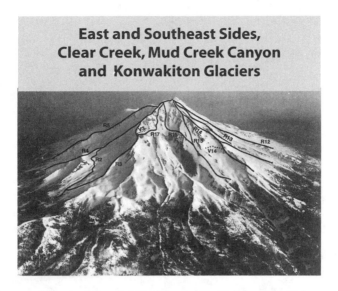

**East and Southeast Sides,
Clear Creek, Mud Creek Canyon
and Konwakiton Glaciers**

The southeast side of Mt. Shasta is distinguished by a very broad, gentle shoulder between the Konwakiton Glacier and the great cleft of Mud Creek canyon, and the Wintun Glacier. This gradual slope was noticed early in Shasta's climbing history, and it became popular because of its ease. This was the way Old Jump Up, the first horse to stand atop Mt. Shasta, made his notable climb in the very early 1900s. Evidence of an old trail is often seen in times of light snow. High camps of the early climbers are still found, occasionally complete with neat, small stacks of sun-bleached firewood carried above timberline before the advent of today's ultralight camp stoves.

Route 15   CLEAR CREEK

DIFFICULTY: 1 (F)

ACCESS: Clear Creek Trailhead

CAMPSITES: Clear Creek, Pilgrim Creek's many intermittent meadows and springs

TIME: 1 day

From one of several excellent base camp sites between Mud Creek and Clear Creek, the broad, gradual slope of the climbing route is very evident, resembling a gently tilted isosceles triangle. In spring

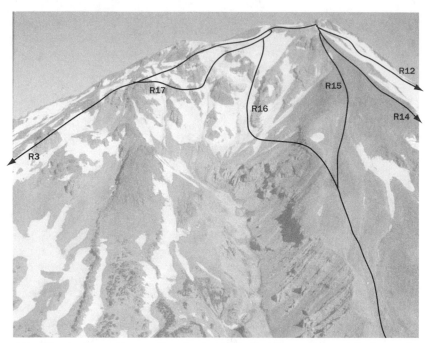

Mt. Shasta from the southeast, showing the Konwakiton Glacier and upper Clear Creek route

and early summer, abundant snow allows an easy climb. However, the southern exposure causes the snowpack to melt rapidly, leaving unpleasant talus and sand. In late summer you must try to find a route that links snowfields together to bypass most of the talus. At 13,000 feet avoid steep chutes dropping off on either side of the climbing route, to the Konwakiton and the Wintun glaciers. This pleasing route ends on the broad summit snowfield just west of the summit pinnacle.

Descend via the climbing route.

Route 16   KONWAKITON GLACIER FROM THE EAST

DIFFICULTY: 3 (AD+)

ACCESS: Clear Creek trailheads

CAMPSITES: Clear Creek, Pilgrim Creek's many intermittent meadows and springs

TIME: 1+ to 2 days

The Konwakiton ("Muddy One," in the Wintun Indian language) Glacier is one of Shasta's smallest glaciers, extending down only to about 12,000 feet. The glacier lies at the head of Mt. Shasta's most immense gorge, Mud Creek Canyon, and only the imagination can ponder the scale of the geologic and glacial events that shaped this huge chasm. Here is some of the steepest and most rugged terrain on Mt. Shasta.

The best approach to the climbing route is via a traverse from the Clear Creek route. Begin the traverse at an elevation near or above waterfalls emanating from the glacier's foot. Rockfall can be a serious problem on this route. Take great care on the approach, as the sun can soften the rock's frozen mortar from above. A vertical rock ridge divides the glacier; you can pass left of this ridge to gain immediate entrance to the steep icefall, or pass the ridge on its right to avoid the icefall altogether. There are many variations on the glacier—from steep, difficult ice to challenging mixed climbing on rock ribs. The slope of the glacier decreases near its apex. Climb northeast to the summit snowfield and continue to the summit pinnacle.

Descend via the Clear Creek route (R15).

Route 17　KONWAKITON GLACIER FROM THE SOUTH

DIFFICULTY: 3 (AD+)

ACCESS: Everitt Memorial Highway

CAMPSITES: Panther Meadow, old Ski Bowl lodge parking area

TIME: 1 to 2 days

From Sargents Ridge you can establish a high camp on the north side of Shastarama Point or at the base of the Mud Creek Glacier. Approach the Konwakiton Glacier from the southwest. The easiest approach will be dictated by current conditions. You can avoid the icefall by climbing steep gullies on the left. When adequate snow cover is present and loose rocks are cemented well in place, it's convenient to traverse below the icefall to direct ascent lines east of the rock ridge dividing the glacier.

Descend via Sargents Ridge.

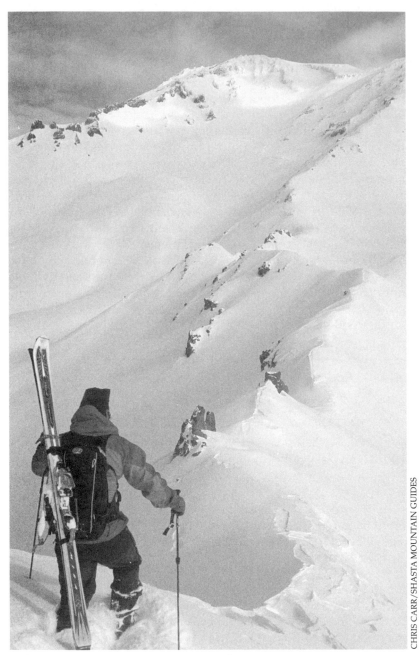

Ski mountaineering on Green Butte Ridge

CHRIS CARR/SHASTA MOUNTAIN GUIDES

114

5

SKIING, SNOWBOARDING, AND SKI-TOURING

VAST GLACIERS AND SNOWFIELDS, immense vertical drops, and plentiful winter snowfall have long attracted skiers and snowboarders to Mt. Shasta. Indeed, one popular backcountry ski magazine has referred to Mt. Shasta as *"one of the best backcountry ski mountains on the planet!"* During winter, skiers and snowboarders of all abilities, as well as snowshoers and winter campers, can find endless opportunities for recreation on the mountain. Even during the height of a storm, enjoyable skiing and snowboarding awaits within the protected forests below timberline. During spring and early summer many of the climbing routes can be combined with an exciting partial or complete descent on skis or snowboard—beginning from as high as the summit. Favorable snow conditions often allow descents of more than 6000 vertical feet!

At the beginning of the 20th century, skis were used almost exclusively for transportation, not recreation. But some of the hardy early pioneers began to discover adventure and fun on the downhill runs. In the 1920s and 30s skiers flocked to Snowman's Hill, on Mt. Shasta's gentle southern slopes, to schuss and watch ski jumping contests among some of North America's finest skiers. Southern Pacific Railroad had special weekend trains from San Francisco to this popular ski destination. Historic Snowman's Hill remains today as a Forest Service-maintained snowplay area.

The earliest ski descents of Mt. Shasta were made in the 1920s and 30s, remarkable events considering the archaic equipment of the time, and the magnitude and steepness of the mountain. In 1925, Swiss mountaineers skied as far as the saddle between Shasta and Shastina. In the 1930s, a group of Yale ski team members, themselves intimidated by Mt. Shasta's scale, estimated that "'The

115

drop from the summit to Horse Camp can be done easily, by an experienced man, in five minutes!"

In April 1932, Hvalor Hvalstad, Steffen Trogstad, and Tex Red, professional ski jumpers who came to Mt. Shasta to compete at Snowman's Hill, made the first ski descent from Shasta's summit. The descent took one hour and fifteen minutes, and for amusement they made a small ski hill and jumped over the cabin at Horse Camp! The first solo ski descent was made by Olympic ski coach, Otto Steiner, in 1936. Today, skiers and snowboarders come from afar for Mt. Shasta's world-class descents and ski-touring.

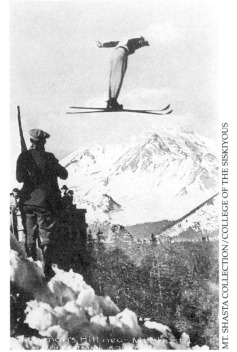

Ski jumping on Snowman's Hill, circa 1937

In this chapter we describe the range of ski and snowboarding possibilities on Mt. Shasta. Ski mountaineering and all backcountry skiing require knowledge of technique, proper equipment, and the ability to be self-sufficient. Preparation for and experience with various snow conditions, weather conditions, and avalanche dangers should be considered *de rigueur*, as there are no cookbook formulas or shortcuts for avoiding potential dangers and hazards on Mt. Shasta—or on any other mountain.

Although several Shasta glaciers offer moderate descents, they still require proper glacier travel technique, ability, and equipment. The most crucial hazard that backcountry skiers and snowboarders have to contend with is avalanches. Beginners who stick to meadows and gentle slopes in the forest have little to worry about, but when you enter the realm of backcountry skiing, ski mountaineering, and snowboarding you enter the realm of potential avalanches. Avalanche forecasting is a fascinating subject, and you are urged to seek instruction. Many excellent texts on the subject are available, as are classes, seminars, and avalanche-transceiver training. Because Mt. Shasta receives plenty of snowfall, most (but not all) avalanches on Shasta are "direct-action" avalanches, which occur during storms or soon after, as a result of new snow loading the slopes.

Current snow and weather conditions can always be obtained locally in order to help you plan and prepare for an outing. Phone numbers for 24-hour weather and climbing information, as well as informative websites, are listed at the end of the "Weather" chapter in this book. The website www.shastaavalanche.org has daily postings.

Ski and snowboard routes can be described only in general terms. Terrain, snow conditions, weather, visibility, and potential avalanche danger vary seasonally, and even daily. Certain routes and tours are best at certain seasons, as indicated below.

Skiing and snowboarding on Mt. Shasta may be divided into four general categories:

I.   **A ski or snowboard descent in conjunction with one of the climbing routes.** This may be the conclusion of a summit climb, or skiing and snowboarding may be the objective.

II. **Highway winter access.** The best access for beginner/intermediate skiers and snowboarders, and for access to some selected advanced runs, is Everitt Memorial Highway on Shasta's southwest side. This highway is plowed regularly as far as Bunny Flat.

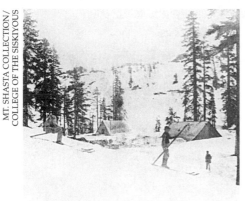

MT. SHASTA COLLECTION/
COLLEGE OF THE SISKIYOUS

III. **Ski-in base camps.** Many excellent skiing areas require a long skiing approach, but a base camp in a wilderness setting makes the effort worthwhile. Access to such places via gravel roads varies with the season.

IV. **Lift-serviced and cross-country ski areas.** Mt. Shasta Board & Ski Park and Nordic Center both operate on a regular schedule throughout the winter.

Early skiers on Mt. Shasta, using alpenstocks to control their speed

In addition, we describe:

V. Castle Lake highway access, Mt. Eddy, and the west side of Strawberry Valley.

VI. Mt. Shasta Ski Circumnavigation.

SKIING AND SNOWBOARDING: THE CLIMBING ROUTES

Many of the climbing routes on Shasta are excellent ski routes as well. With a little added equipment and preparation, these climbing routes can become exciting ski or snowboard descents. Access, route descriptions and other information appear in detail in the "Climbing" chapter. The following is a sequential listing—clockwise around Mt. Shasta from Avalanche Gulch—of the best climb/ski routes, along with special comments as they apply.

Key to Ski and Snowboard Routes

Access: The best approach, road or otherwise, at various seasons.

Season: The time of year for the best skiing and snowboarding of the route or area.

Level: Degree of difficulty of skiing in area. (We've tried to balance the ratings between cross-country/telemark, snowboard, and downhill equipment. On the more difficult descents, the skiing will tend to be a little harder than the rating if you're using cross-country gear, a little easier if you're using randonee or downhill gear.)

🔺 means previously recorded avalanche activity

Route 1 🔺 **TRADITIONAL JOHN MUIR/ AVALANCHE GULCH**

SEASON: Spring to early summer

LEVEL: Advanced

Avalanche Gulch, the immense, open bowl on Shasta's southwest flank, offers nearly unlimited skiing possibilities. For those desiring a descent from the actual summit, this route has the most consistent snow conditions, although the reaches above the Red Banks often have poor quality and/or sparse snow cover, as well as icy sections. Choose your line carefully through or around the Red Banks, as this series of chimneys can be difficult to negotiate, and there is no dishonor in taking the board(s) off here. The skiing and boarding is best on "corn" snow.

Variation 1a ⏿ **Left of Heart**

SEASON: Spring to early summer

Level: Advanced to Expert

This steep variation avoids the Red Banks when they're lacking enough skiable snow. and for pure exposure this run is one of the most exciting on Mt. Shasta. The Red Banks headwall varies seasonally, but you can expect pitches up to and exceeding 40 degrees.

Route 2 ⏿ **OLD SKI BOWL**

SEASON: Spring to early summer

LEVEL: Intermediate to Advanced

This bowl is pleasant and scenic. It's impractical to ski this route starting from above 10,000 feet because of steep rock cliffs, but the route can be connected by traverse to Route 1 for maximum vertical drop. Snowmobiles are allowed in this area, and they are not uncommon.

Route 4 ⏿ **GREEN BUTTE RIDGE**

SEASON: Late winter to early spring

LEVEL: Intermediate to Advanced

This ridge offers access to several other bowls, and also can be connected to Route 1. If you're itching to get above tree line but conditions are avalanche-prone, this route often has a much lower hazard.

Variation 5 ⬣ **West Face Gully**

SEASON: Spring to early summer

LEVEL: Advanced to Expert

This steep, open gully is a candidate for the "extreme" category, but sun-softened spring snow can bring it into the range of many skiers. The run includes a continuous fall-line shot for 4000 feet, making it one of Mt. Shasta's most exciting descents. The upper headwall can be steep, but moving west lessens the severity of this short section.

Route 6 ⬣ **CASCADE GULCH**

SEASON: Spring to early summer

LEVEL: Intermediate to Advanced

This very delightful, curving, open bowl allows a moderate, traversing descent from Shastina to Horse Camp.

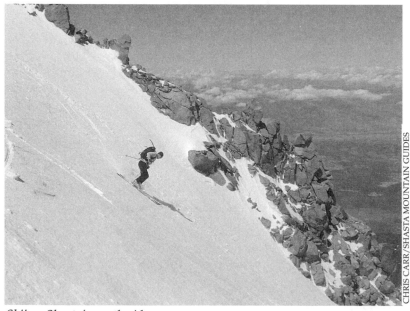

Skiing Shasta's north side

Route 7 ⚠ WHITNEY GLACIER

SEASON: Late winter to early summer
LEVEL: Intermediate to Advanced

With adequate snow cover the vast lower glacier is excellent for skiing, and it provides access for winter and spring ascents of the upper glacier.

Variation 7b ⚠ Whitney-Bolam Ridge

SEASON: Late winter to early spring
LEVEL: Advanced

This ridge is an excellent ski descent when there is ample snow.

Route 8 ⚠ BOLAM GLACIER FROM THE NORTHWEST

SEASON: Late winter to early spring
LEVEL: Intermediate to Advanced

The Bolam's lack of serious crevasses makes it Shasta's best glacier to ski.

Route 9 ⚠ BOLAM GLACIER FROM THE NORTHEAST

SEASON: Late winter to early summer
LEVEL: Intermediate to Advanced

The North Gate road and trailhead, often open by late spring, makes this one of the earliest-opening ski descents apart from the south side.

Variation 9a ⚠ Bolam Gully

SEASON: Spring
LEVEL: Advanced to Expert

The Bolam Gully is another ski descent route in the "extreme" category.

Route 10 Ⓐ HOTLUM-BOLAM RIDGE

SEASON: Spring to early summer
LEVEL: Advanced

Above 13,000 feet the ridge proper may not be skiable because of exposed rocks and wind-scoured snow and ice, but the snowfields on either side of the ridge remain in skiable condition remarkably late into summer, and can be connected in many ways for superb ski descents.

Route 11 Ⓐ HOTLUM GLACIER

SEASON: Spring
LEVEL: Advanced

The Hotlum Glacier is not especially steep, but it can be difficult to ski because of the large icefalls and a maze of crevasses. However, careful route finding will reach excellent ski terrain.

Route 12 Ⓐ HOTLUM-WINTUN RIDGE

SEASON: Late winter to early summer
LEVEL: Intermediate to Advanced

This route is considered by many to be one of the finest descents on Mt. Shasta, and is usually one of the longest-lasting snow slopes on Shasta, often skiable through the summer, or until sun cups become too large. During favorable snow conditions, it is possible to ski off the actual summit by this route, and the following route, the Wintun Glacier.

The upper sections can be steep with wind-scoured snow, but the eastern exposure often produces excellent "corn" snow. Minimal crevasse hazard makes for a very enjoyable and consistent descent. The roads to the trailhead are usually inaccessible until early or mid-June, depending on the winter snowpack, but this descent is worthy of an early ski-approach.

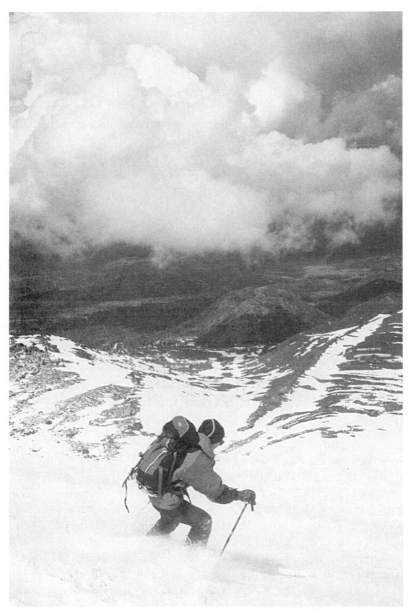

Skiing Hotlum-Bolam Ridge

Route 13 Ⓐ WINTUN GLACIER

SEASON: Spring to early summer
LEVEL: Advanced

The upper reaches of the glacier are excellent skiing, and they can be connected with Route 12 for a long descent.

The following two routes are spring favorites, offering broad, wide skiing terrain with moderate slopes.

Route 14 Ⓐ WINTUN RIDGE

SEASON: Late winter to spring
LEVEL: Intermediate to Advanced

Route 15 Ⓐ CLEAR CREEK

SEASON: Late winter to spring
LEVEL: Intermediate to Advanced

WINTER ACCESS:
EVERITT MEMORIAL HIGHWAY

In 1912 local citizens decided that a wagon road from the town of Sisson to Horse Camp was necessary to promote tourism. Work was begun on the popularly called "Mt. Shasta Snowline Highway" in 1927 and completed all the way to Panther Meadows by 1940. In 1934 the uncompleted highway was renamed "The John Samuel Everitt Memorial Highway" in honor of the supervisor of the Shasta National Forest who had died on August 25, 1934, fighting a fire on Shasta's southern flanks.

Paved in 1956, the road is now known as Everitt Memorial Highway. Complete with milestones and elevation markers along its 14-mile length, the highway was plowed regularly throughout the winter during the heyday of the Mt. Shasta Ski Bowl. Since the Ski Bowl ceased operation in 1978, Siskiyou County road crews now plow only to the 11-mile point, at Bunny Flat. The remaining 3 miles of the road remain beneath snow, usually through June, but the road is still easy to follow and it makes for an enjoyable ski tour.

The early designers of the highway had probably never seen skis when they began planning the road, but their design was fortuitous: Everitt Memorial Highway allows access to some of the finest and most varied skiing found anywhere on Shasta. There is parking at Bunny Flat (11 miles), Sand Flat (10 miles) and the Wagon Camp turnout, or switchback (7 miles). Snowmobiles are allowed below Everitt Memorial Highway up to the old Ski Bowl.

They are also allowed to travel in the bowl itself. Always use caution when these vehicles are nearby, or when sharing a narrow track with them.

The following areas are arranged in descending progression, from greater to lesser elevation, along Everitt Memorial Highway from the old Ski Bowl, and continue clockwise from the highway around the mountain.

UNPLOWED EVERITT HIGHWAY, BUNNY FLAT TO OLD SKI BOWL

LEVEL: Beginner to Intermediate

OTHER ACTIVITY: Snowshoeing

The gently contoured Everitt Highway, under snow its last 3 miles from Bunny Flat to Panther Meadow, is easy to follow as it winds through stately Shasta red fir trees. This is an excellent short tour with an easy return.

OLD SKI BOWL ⊘

LEVEL: Intermediate to Advanced

In the days of the old ski area, the two sides of this large, open cirque were identified as the "West Bowl" and the "East Bowl." The west bowl, adjacent to precipitous Green Butte, is steep and challenging; the east bowl is more rolling and gentle.

TOUR TO SOUTH GATE MEADOWS/SQUAW VALLEY ⬠

LEVEL: Intermediate to Advanced

OTHER ACTIVITY: Snow camping

From the bottom of the Ski Bowl cirque, traverse east through an obvious notch in Sargents Ridge. Continue through The Gate, the pass between Red Butte and the mountain, and into the beautiful hemlock forests of South Gate Meadows/Squaw Valley. Continue to ski farther east for outstanding winter views of the Konwakiton Glacier and Mud Creek Canyon.

PANTHER MEADOWS

LEVEL: Beginner to Intermediate

OTHER ACTIVITIES: Snowshoeing, snow camping

Below the old Ski Bowl and just west of Gray Butte are the gentle rolling hills and forest of Panther Meadows. Close proximity to parking at Bunny Flat makes the meadows a desirable destination for snow camping or ski touring. A pleasant side trip, all downhill, is to ski 2.5 miles cross-country south to Mt. Shasta Board & Ski Park. Pre-arrange a shuttle or a pick-up for this variation.

WAGON CAMP

LEVEL: Intermediate

From Panther Meadows traverse west, parallel to and below Everitt Memorial Highway, through forest and open slopes. Finish at the Wagon Camp switchback, a convenient shuttle point.

GRAY BUTTE NORTHWEST FACE ⬠

LEVEL: Advanced

Gray Butte is the steep hill bordering the southeast edge of Panther Meadows. The best approach to ski the north face of the butte is via the ridge on the left (N) of the north face.

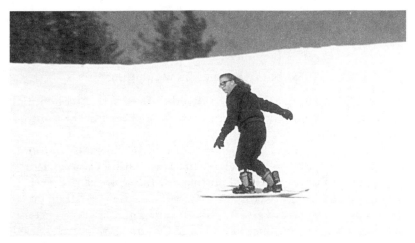

Snowboarding Broadway

POWDER BOWL AND SUN BOWL ◬

LEVEL: Intermediate to Advanced

Powder Bowl and Sun Bowl are the two very distinct, above-timberline bowls between Green Butte and Bunny Flat, Sun Bowl being the westernmost. The easiest approach is via Green Butte Ridge from Bunny Flat. The lower parts of these bowls may be reached from several points along the unplowed Everitt Memorial Highway track. These two bowls offer some of the finest early spring snow on Shasta, as long as avalanche risk is minimal.

BROADWAY ◬

LEVEL: Intermediate to Advanced

The wide lower half of Green Butte Ridge is called Broadway. The skiing here is excellent when sufficient snow covers some very large rocks.

BUNNY FLAT AREA

LEVEL: Beginner to Intermediate

OTHER ACTIVITIES: Snowshoeing, snow camping

Bunny Flat, at the end of the plowed part of Everitt Memorial Highway, is parking area, staging area and hub for ski tours in every direction.

The most popular half-day ski tour on Mt. Shasta is undoubtedly the short jaunt to the Sierra Club Foundation cabin at Horse Camp. From Bunny Flat head north a few hundred yards, passing through an obvious break in the near ridge to the west, then gradually climbing northwest. Yellow metal triangles—old license plates—on trees mark this ski trail. A 25 foot metal rain tower, used by the Forest Service as a rain collecting gauge, marks the two-thirds point of the route. The cabin is always unlocked, and it makes a wonderful winter base camp or a place for lunch and socializing.

You can also ski to Sand Flat or Wagon Camp from Bunny Flat, shuttle back up Everitt Memorial Highway, and repeat the run.

HORSE CAMP AREA AND BEYOND ⬢

LEVEL: Beginner, Intermediate, Advanced

OTHER ACTIVITY: Snowshoeing, snow camping

The Sierra Club Foundation cabin is an excellent base camp for skiing in the cabin's own backyard: the immense Avalanche Gulch basin. North of the cabin are advanced-level bowls, Cascade Gulch and Hidden Valley.

HORSE CAMP TO MCBRIDE SPRINGS ⬢

LEVEL: Intermediate to Advanced

This is one of the best descents on the southwest slope of Shasta. From the Sierra Club Foundation cabin, traverse north a quarter mile and follow the slopes on the south side of Cascade Gulch until you meet Everitt Memorial Highway near the McBride Springs campground. This ski descent is more than 4 miles long and drops more than 4000 vertical feet.

SAND FLAT AREA

LEVEL: Beginner to Intermediate

OTHER ACTIVITIES: Snowshoeing, snow camping

Sand Flat is a beautiful open meadow with postcard-perfect views of upper Mt. Shasta. The meadow can be reached by a 0.5 mile ski-in on one of two easy-to-follow snow-covered roads. There is a parking area at the upper road (10.2 milepost and SAND FLAT

SPECIAL EXTRA: Diller Canyon ⊘

SEASON: Spring to summer

LEVEL: Advanced to Expert

Diller Canyon is the very large and unmistakable cleft in the west face of Shastina. It was named after USGS geologist Joseph Diller, who conducted studies on Shasta during the 1880s. Throughout the winter, strong jet-stream-velocity north winds carry enormous quantities of snow from Shastina's flanks to the lee (S) side of the canyon, where it remains throughout the summer. Although this is not a particularly worthy climbing route, as a ski descent it is one of the longest and most exciting on Shasta. For the expert skier, this one should not be missed. And for snowboarders, consider this the largest and longest half-pipe on the planet!

Access to Diller Canyon can be a problem because of rough dirt roads; a truck with ample clearance or a 4-wheel-drive vehicle is necessary. Drive up Everitt Memorial Highway 3.6 miles to a dirt road on the left marked BLACK BUTTE TRAILHEAD. Follow this dirt road 0.8 mile, then turn east on another dirt road. Follow this road as it curves north, then west, then north again to as high as possible along Shastina's flank. (Disrepair and constant additions to this maze of logging roads cause yearly changes to access direction. If in doubt, follow the line of least resistance to as high as possible; the hike to Diller Canyon is scenic and not very long.)

sign), and another at the lower road, about 0.6 mile down Everitt Memorial Highway from Upper Sand Flat Road and its parking area. The upper road is nearly flat; the lower one is steeper but more fun to ski down. The Forest Service has placed signs on the trees to mark several easy scenic tours within the area. A cross-country ski-trail map for Sand Flat is available at the Mt. Shasta Ranger Station.

RED FIR FLAT

LEVEL: Beginner

OTHER ACTIVITIES: Snowshoeing, snow camping

Located just below the lower road to Sand Flat, the gentle terrain of Red Fir Flat is especially suited for beginners.

SKI-IN BASE CAMPS: WILDERNESS SKIING

A true winter delight is skiing into a plateau or a protected valley, establishing a comfortable base camp, and then skiing untracked terrain during this most magical time in the wilderness. Mt. Shasta has several such secret spots. Keep in mind that the only limiting factor is your imagination. A guidebook may be useful, but a sense of adventure is the key. A little extra effort may be required to get to the chosen areas, but the reward is wilderness skiing at its finest. Following are a few of the best areas.

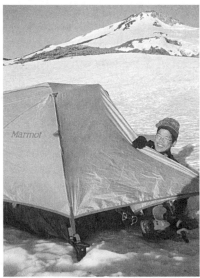

The north and northeast sides of Shasta sometimes experience unusual winter weather effects: a cold stillness descends and dry powder snow remains in the valleys and the gullies for weeks on end. When the Military Pass

Waking up below the Hotlum Glacier

and Andesite roads are open, access to the North Gate and to the Inconstance, Gravel and Brewer Creek drainages is afforded. Excellent snow is usually found here.

Similar excellent snow conditions can often be found on Shasta's east flanks, but access depends upon how far you can first drive up Pilgrim Creek Road. A long ski-in to base camp is usually necessary, but the terrain is gentle. The Cold, Pilgrim, Ash and Clear Creek drainages offer the best snow.

LIFT-SERVICED AND COMMERCIAL SKI AREAS

Mt. Shasta has a long history of downhill skiing, going back to the early 1930s when the "Mount Shasta Snowmen" ski club was organized. Snowman's Hill, at the crest of Hwy. 89 between the towns of McCloud and Mount Shasta, was a 90-meter ski jump considered to be one of the best ski-jumping hills in North America during the 1930s. Southern Pacific Railroad had special weekend ski trains from the San Francisco Bay Area to Snowman's Hill, and several ski-jumping championships were held there. The Forest Service still maintains this area for snowplay, sliding, and sledding.

When Everitt Memorial Highway was completed in 1940, several plans for ski lifts on the mountain were proposed. These different proposals included, at various times, lifts from the town of Mount Shasta to the top of the mountain! The old Mt. Shasta Ski Bowl, located above Panther Meadow, operated from 1958 until 1978. The Mt. Shasta Board & Ski Park, below Panther Meadow and Gray Butte, opened in 1985. It has three triple chairs and a surface lift, complete lodge facilities, ski school and night skiing—all on groomed trails serving beginners to experts. In addition, it has a telemark program and instruction, and a Nordic ski area with over 40 kilometers of groomed trails, lodge facilities and trailside warming huts, and lessons.

The Mt. Shasta Board & Ski Park also offers a summer program that includes scenic chairlift rides, mountain biking, guided nature hikes, natural history exhibits, and various special events.

THE EDDYS, CASTLE LAKE AND BEYOND

The "Eddys" refers to the mountains across the valley to the west of Mt. Shasta, dominated by 9025-foot Mt. Eddy. The Klamath, Siskiyou and Scott mountains all meet in this area, which is very old geologically compared to Mt. Shasta. If you're adventurous, spectacular mountain scenery, hidden backcountry bowls, and possibilities for exploration abound in the Eddys. The Castle Lake Road, snowplowed as far as the lake on an irregular basis, is a good departure point. A special backcountry ski-touring map for this area is available at the Fifth Season outdoor shop in Mount Shasta; other maps are available at the District Ranger office.

MT. SHASTA SKI CIRCUMNAVIGATION

Mt. Shasta's quintessential ski tour is for advanced and expert backcountry skiers. The general rule of thumb is to remain near timberline, although many variations are possible.

A clockwise direction of travel is best, usually starting from the Sierra Club Foundation cabin at Horse Camp. This starting point is especially advised because if the nearby northwest flanks of Shastina have been scoured of snow by the wind, as they often have been, skiers can easily backtrack to the cabin.

A counterclockwise course could bring you to the northwest side of Shastina several days after beginning the trip, with no convenient escape route if lack of snow prevented a skiing return to the cabin. Some additional caveats: You can cross Ash Creek canyon either above or below the falls. Going above the falls entails elevation gain, but offers an easy canyon crossing. Going low offers the protection of the forest, but a steeper canyon to cross. Mud Creek canyon should be crossed in the vicinity of its confluence with Clear Creek. Any higher crossing is steeper and longer; a lower crossing means additional gorges to contend with and considerable elevation to regain.

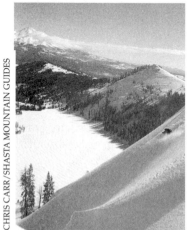

This circumnavigation is an unforgettable ski trip on a great mountain. Needless to say, careful preparations, heavy-duty equipment, and self-sufficiency are necessary. You should plan on 4 or 5 days for the ski circumnavigation of Mt. Shasta.

Fresh powder above frozen Castle Lake

CHRIS CARR/SHASTA MOUNTAIN GUIDES

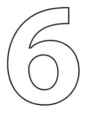

WATER ACTIVITIES

MT. SHASTA is a gigantic, porous mass of volcanic material that absorbs water from glaciers, surface snow and rain like a huge sponge. The porous rock within the mountain's mass acts like a giant reservoir—an aquifer—slowly releasing its water through a number of springs surrounding the mountain. The temperature of the water is constant throughout the year, and the quantity and quality of the water are very high.

The Sacramento, Shasta and McCloud rivers are all directly fed from the Mt. Shasta aquifer. There are three other major rivers nearby, and although not within the Mt. Shasta watershed, they offer some of the finest whitewater in the west. The Klamath, Scott, and Salmon rivers offer excellent boating, from class I (easiest) to class V (expert), on runs as short as a few hours or as long as several days. Commercial river rafters and professional guides are available for all of these rivers, and you can obtain their listings from the various district rangers and outdoor shops. We've listed some of the best whitewater runs, along with information on put-ins and take-outs, difficulty, hazards, and the most interesting sections.

BOATING, RAFTING AND KAYAKING

The Sacramento and McCloud rivers, within Mt. Shasta's watershed influence, will give you excellent whitewater thrills throughout the spring and summer. The McCloud stretch begins at the lower falls in Fowler's campground east of the town of McCloud off Hwy. 89. The river passes through lush, old-growth forests and ends at Lake McCloud, where a boat ramp facilitates take-out and shuttles. The McCloud is not open to commercial rafting companies or outfitters, so you'll have to tackle this gem without help.

The upper Sacramento River canyon offers a cornucopia of exciting whitewater runs from Dunsmuir to Shasta Lake. There are numerous points for put-in and take-out, and you'll find several surprise views of Mt. Shasta to be unforgettable. Plan for up to a full day. The Sacramento River is open to commercial river outfitters; you can obtain current listings and brochures of these concessionaires from an outdoor shop or the district ranger offices.

THE SACRAMENTO RIVER

South Fork

The headwaters of the Sacramento River begin in the city park of the town of Mt. Shasta. Coursing over 50 miles to Shasta Lake, the Sacramento has a plethora of sections from class I to class V that will satisfy everyone from relaxing rafters to squirt-boat experts.

One of the most exciting sections is South Fork, just above Lake Siskiyou west of the town of Mount Shasta. This is a class IV-V section with a steep gradient, frequent large boulders, and occasional logs from the heavy runoff of winter snows. You can put in at the first green bridge above the lake, about 4 miles, or venture farther upstream for even more serious paddling. This exciting run finishes at the tranquil water of Lake Siskiyou, where you can take out

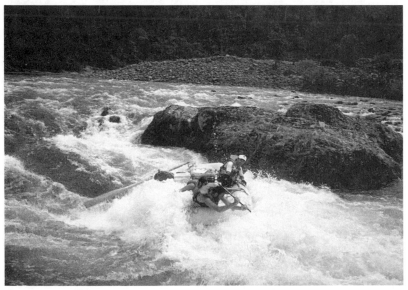

Sacramento River

at the campground boat ramp, or the dam at the southeast end of the lake.

Box Canyon

Box Canyon is the narrow, steep-walled ravine immediately below the dam at the southeast end of Lake Siskiyou. This enjoyable class III-IV run can be a short afternoon paddle to nearby take-out, or a longer journey to the historic railroad town of Dunsmuir and beyond.

The put-in is difficult and requires care. The trail starts at the east end of the dam and winds along the edge of a golf course for a few hundred yards to a fork. Take the right branch and descend a steep trail along a cliff band. A short steel ladder and fixed rope end at the water. Once in the canyon, the lush views are spectacular. The rapids are well-defined with plenty of pools and eddies in which to linger. After 2.5 miles, you can take-out at the Cantara fishing access, or continue 4 more miles to Dunsmuir, where a convenient take-out area exists at the I-5 bridge. The section from Cantara to Dunsmuir is best during high water.

Sims to Gibson or Pollard Flat

The section of the upper Sacramento River from Sims, a few miles below Castle Crags State Park, to take-outs at Gibson (5 miles) and Pollard Flat (6.5 miles), offers mellow class III whitewater with moderate excitement and excellent scenery. The put-ins and take-outs are I-5 exits which lie east of the freeway. There are many large pools and drops, as well as gentle eddies. Much of this section of the river zigs and zags underneath the railroad tracks which parallel the river throughout the entirety of the run.

THE UPPER MCCLOUD RIVER

The McCloud River, fed directly from Mt. Shasta south- and east-side glaciers, is one of the clearest and coldest rivers in northern California. This class III+ river passes through one of the most beautiful and lush primal forests at the foot of Mt. Shasta, and the 6-mile section to the McCloud reservoir is continually entertaining.

The put-in is at Fowler campground, just off Hwy. 89 about 6 miles east of the town of McCloud. Signs at the campground mark river access. After about 0.75 mile, the river doubles in size at Big Springs, a beautiful wall of water gushing from artesian springs in the lava rock. Be on the lookout for fallen trees and snags occasionally spanning the river. The location of these obstructions varies from year to year depending on the severity of the previous winter. During the last third of the run you'll be surprised to see fantastic fairytale chalets and castles along the shore of the Hearst property. Remember to stay in your boats so as not to trespass on this private land. After you reach the McCloud reservoir, there is a 2.5 mile paddle to the take-out at Tarantula Gulch boat ramp. This take-out is reached by driving 12 miles southeast on Squaw Valley Road from the town of McCloud. Plan for a full day for this outstanding, scenic river.

THE SCOTT RIVER

Kelsey Creek to Scott Bar

The Scott River, beginning in the Marble Mountain Wilderness and Salmon–Trinity Alps, is a member of the National Wild and Scenic Rivers System. This excellent 10-mile class III to class V section is often split into two runs, Kelsey Creek to Townsend Gulch (4 miles) and Townsend Gulch to Scott Bar (6 miles). The upper stretch is more popular and has the largest and most difficult rapids. The largest is known as "Whitehouse," and is overlooked by Scott River Lodge on the left. After another 0.3 mile, you come to Tompkins Creek rapid, requiring maneuvering through swift water and sizable boulders. The Townsend Gulch take-out is another 0.75 mile downstream on the left.

Townsend Gulch to Scott Bar is somewhat easier than the upper stretches of the Scott River as the canyon widens and the rapids begin to lessen in severity. The take-out for this section is at the bridge at Scott Bar.

THE SALMON RIVER

The Salmon River, located in Siskiyou County's northwest corner, is in an extremely remote location. Driving through the canyons of the Salmon is like driving through the Swiss Alps without the civilized feel of Europe. Narrow, winding roads, sometimes clinging to cliffs, make getting to the put-in, or just running the shuttle, an adventure in itself. The remoteness, and the required preparations, are well worth the effort, for the Salmon River, while almost completely devoid of après-trip amenities, offers some of California's most exciting whitewater amidst stunning scenery.

South Fork—Matthews Creek
Campground to Forks of Salmon

This is a delightful 10-mile class III to III+ run over a gravel and granite streambed. There is one rapid of class IV difficulty about 3.5 miles from the put-in. It can be easily scouted from river level along the right bank. After another 0.5 mile is Methodist Creek bridge, which is an alternative put-in for those not wanting to contend with the class IV rapid just upstream. This put-in shortens the run to 6.5 miles. The river continues on for about 1.5 miles at class III difficulty before crossing under the shuttle road. For the next 3 miles the river widens and mellows. There is a 2-mile class III finale to the take-out, about 0.5 mile below the confluence of the South and North Forks of the Salmon River.

North Fork—Little North Fork
Campground to Forks of Salmon

From the put-in, there are continuous class III-IV long, rocky rapids with abrupt, sometimes surprise drops. For the first few miles, the canyon is fairly wide with cobblestone-sized rocks and mine tailings. During the last few miles above the Forks, the river enters a narrower gorge with numerous rock falls forming the rapids. There are appropriate take-outs before this difficult section, but they must be scouted carefully while driving the shuttle. If you float all the way down to Forks of Salmon, the take-out is the same as for the South Fork run.

Salmon River (Main Stem)—
Nordheimer Creek to Salmon River Bridge

The put-in for this outstanding 10-mile stretch of class IV to V river is nearly 4 miles downstream from Forks of Salmon at the site of what was formerly known as Bloomer Falls. This extreme, twisting drop was the most difficult section of the river. In 1983 the Department of Fish and Game dynamited the falls to improve the migration route for salmon swimming upstream to spawn, thus reducing Bloomers to a class III zig-zag. Some boaters divide this stretch into two separate runs, ending the first section at Butler

Creek after 6.5 miles. Butler Creek to the take-out at Salmon River Bridge is about 4 more miles. First-timers on these two sections of river should consider boating with persons already familiar with the runs.

THE KLAMATH RIVER

The Klamath River, second in size in California only to the Sacramento River, begins east of Crater Lake in Oregon, courses through the Cascade Range and numerous lesser mountain ranges, finally reaching the Pacific Ocean south of Crescent City, California. The Klamath runs unimpeded from Iron Gate damn near the California-Oregon border, offering boaters journeys as long as a week.

Tree of Heaven Campground
to Gottville River Access

This 7.5 mile, class II+ to III- section begins just a few miles west on highway 96 from I-5, and is an excellent training run with little in the way of threatening rapids or obstacles. The most excitement comes at "schoolhouse drop," 5.75 miles into the run, where the river is split by a large island. There are many excellent play areas in the last third of the run where white water rodeo paddlers practice their elegant and acrobatic moves. Both put-in and take-out are easily found and well-marked with signs along the shuttle road.

John Boyle Powerhouse to Copco

This is a swift, high-volume kayak and raft run that is one of the most exciting on the Klamath River. It is fed by hydroelectric release that assures a boatable flow when many other runs are too low. Late in the summer, however, releases from the powerhouse become sporadic. Be sure and check the latest river flow information before planning a trip on this section.

The put-in is reached by turning south off route 66 in Oregon between mile 42 and 43 at the sign to the John Boyle powerhouse, then continuing 5.5 miles to where the road descends a steep switchback to the river. The run begins with 2 miles of class II and III, followed by 4 miles of easier water. Six miles below the put-in very serious water begins at Caldera rapid. This is followed by

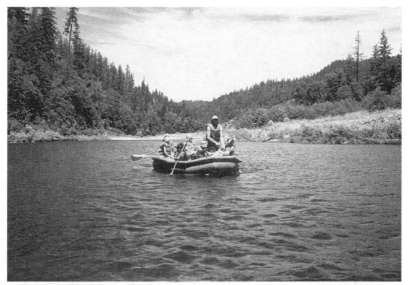

Klamath River

well-named "Satan's Gate," "Hell's Corner," and other large rapids. A little below Stateline Falls the river eases in difficulty and you will encounter the first of several river access points. If you take out at the first access, a BLM fishing access site, you'll eliminate 4 miles of class II paddling from the run. You can also continue to the upper reaches of Copco reservoir and other take-outs.

Appropriate river flows are critical for an enjoyable and safe river trip. River difficulty, water levels, hazards, and obstructions can change dramatically and often. Careful planning and preparation can help make for a safe, enjoyable trip. Be sure to check sources in the "Weather" chapter, as well as www.dreamflows.com and http://cdec.water.ca.gov for current river flow information.

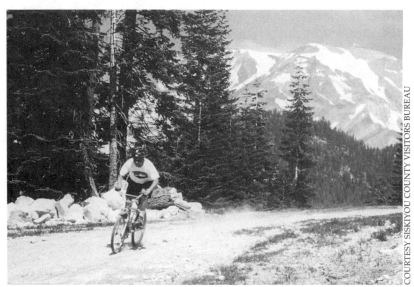

Mountain biker

COURTESY SISKIYOU COUNTY VISITORS BUREAU

7

MOUNTAIN BIKING

MT. SHASTA'S NETWORK of logging roads offers vast backcountry cycling opportunities. To be sure, many roads run through ugly logged areas, and some have frustrating sandy sections, but locals have found that mountain bikes open up a new realm of exploration and adventure on Shasta. The 2005 edition of the topographic map included in this book is designed in part to show these rideable roads Here we suggest a few of the more rewarding trips.

Mountain bikes may be rented at various shops in Mount Shasta. Bike trail maps and route-guides are also available. As in any federal wilderness area, all mechanical transport is barred from the Mt. Shasta Wilderness and the Castle Crags Wilderness, as well as anywhere on the Pacific Crest Trail.

FOREST ROAD 31

From Mt. Shasta Board & Ski Park this main forest road runs east on a good surface and curves north to the east side of the mountain. Here you can join the road to the Clear Creek or to the Brewer Creek trailhead, described in the "Hiking" chapter. You can also meet up with Road 31 by following the driving route to those trailheads, starting on the Pilgrim Creek Road, which branches north off Hwy. 89 east of McCloud.

MCBRIDE RIDES

The most popular and accessible mountain-bike challenges near Mt. Shasta start just north of the town of Mount Shasta, and climb to meet the Everitt Memorial Highway near McBride Springs. An interconnecting network of use trails has developed in this area, offering stimulating rides from intermediate in difficulty to very technical.

Near the start of the Everitt Memorial Highway, just north of Mt. Shasta High School, cross railroad tracks and then promptly turn east (right) onto a dirt road. This road parallels the railroad tracks for some time, but soon you can turn north at any number of trails and old jeep roads. Follow your nose generally north on any of these interconnecting tracks for the climb up, and after about 4-5 miles you'll intersect the Everitt Highway again. Then turn around for the swooping return to a comfortable meal back in town.

The most technical run, recommended for expert riders only, follows the center of a rocky debris flow that spilled through this area during the big floods of New Years 1997. A 5-foot drop near the top of this run highlights the excitement. Other single and dou-ble–track trails offer less intimidating but nevertheless enjoyable descents. Those looking for descent thrills specifically can of course ride up the Everitt Highway to the start of the downhill run, just east of the McBride Springs Campground turnoff.

RAINBOW RIDGE

Local riders enjoy a number of routes that climb up to this ridge, just southwest of the town of Mount Shasta. The jeep track along the crest of this ridge presents excellent views of the Mountain, and includes a variety of both cruising and steep terrain. You may meet an occasional motorcyclist here. From the east you access the ridge from Lake Siskiyou's North Shore Road, and start climbing north onto the ridge about a mile west of the lake. To access the ridge from the northwest, start from Old Stage Road and look for roads heading south from Davis Place road or from the Abrams Lake area. An excellent half-day ride runs across the ridge, con-necting these two access areas. Consult the USGS quadrangles of Mt. Shasta and Mt. Eddy.

THE NORTHERN ARC

This grand, adventurous tour follows quiet, broad back roads around the entire north and east sides of Mt. Shasta, via Military Pass. Although at least one party has completed the trip in one very long day, depending on your end point (arranged with a car shuttle) this is for most people a two-day venture. The route travels outside the range of the map that comes with this book, but the Shasta-Trinity National Forest map is very useful in this case. To avoid midsummer heat, the best times to take this ride are late spring, early summer and fall. From Mount Shasta City, drive north on I-5 to central Weed. At Weed's only stoplight take Hwy. 97 north, and after 12.8 miles turn right (SE) onto Military Pass Road. The classic, full-length ride begins here.

Follow the main road (43N19) over Military Pass, and a few miles after the pass you join with main Forest Road 19. There will be little or no water on this section. Continue south on 19 for about 3 miles, where you'll pass the junction with the road going up to the Brewer Creek trailhead. Just past this junction, veer right (SW) onto Road 31. Continue south on 31, and eventually you'll choose between two main completions. One, you can stay on 31 as it curves in and out of and up and down canyons to the Mt. Shasta Board & Ski Park—and from here you can even continue all the way to the south end of Mount Shasta City, or head due south to meet Hwy. 89 at Snowman's Hill. Alternatively, about 7 miles past the Brewer Creek start of 31, you can turn left (SE) off of 31 onto Road 41N15. This leads downhill in a few miles to pavement at the Pilgrim Creek Road, where you can turn right (SW) and continue on to meet Hwy. 89, 3 miles east of McCloud.

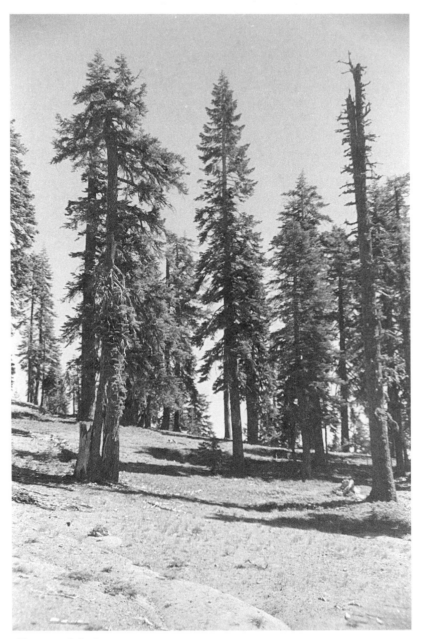

Shasta red fir forest

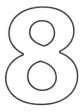

FLORA AND FAUNA

MT. SHASTA stands as a recently created "island" of mountain habitat. Apparently Shasta is a tough home because even though its slopes receive 20-40 feet of snow each winter, most of the slopes are surprisingly dry, even desert-like. Compared to its neighbor volcanoes, Lassen Peak and the Crater Lake volcano, noticeably fewer plant species grow on Shasta. To understand the unusual and relatively Spartan biota of Mt. Shasta, we first have to understand the unusual substrate and the climate.

THE SUBSTRATE

From a hydrologist's point of view, Mt. Shasta is indeed a hollow mountain. The volcanic debris that makes up the mountain is extremely porous, and even the overlying forest soils are too sandy to retain the precious snowmelt. Therefore a large percentage of Mt. Shasta's heavy snowpacks percolates into underground aquifers, and even sizable streams disappear into the ground before they reach low elevations. For the surrounding cities, rivers and lakes, Shasta is a veritable fountain, because the subterranean waters gush out in cold, copious springs all around its perimeter. The plants on the mountain itself, however, are left high and dry. Although other Cascade volcanoes have this percolation effect, none have such extensive dry slopes as Shasta because none have as much porous lava, and those farther north are more covered with glaciers.

THE CLIMATE

At its lookout over both the southern Cascades and California's Central Valley, Mt. Shasta receives an alternation of storms from the north and fair weather from the south. In general, the pattern shifts with the seasons, fair weather dominating in summer and frequent storms blasting the mountain during winter. "Unseasonable surprises" visit every season, though, bringing occasional midsummer storms and long winter sunny spells. Although copious precipitation and sun seem to add up to serendipity for plants, these dramatic "surprises" often make life hard for them.

Mt. Shasta also stands at (and helps form) an east-west climatic divide. On the west, the Pacific Ocean moderates temperatures and pumps moisture into the storms. On the east, the Great Basin contributes drier inland air to Shasta, so the mountain's eastern slopes have colder, drier winters than its western slopes.

These influences are the raw material of Mt. Shasta's climate, but to the life on its slopes the more powerful influence is the way the mountain's mass and its altitude rework weather. Most important among altitude's influences is that when a stormy air mass hits Mt. Shasta and rises upslope, the air expands and cools. Cooler air can hold less moisture, so as storms rise up the mountain they dump ever more rain and snow—up to a point.

Thus, higher elevations have colder temperatures, and they receive more snow and rain—up to a point. Above 8-9000 feet, storms drop less precipitation because the rising air has already given up most of its moisture, and because the thin air at high altitude in general is very dry. Therefore, a typical winter storm on Mt. Shasta will dump increasing rain up to 3-4000 feet, and increasingly heavy snow up to perhaps 9000 feet. Above that we find moderate snowfall, usually accompanied by screaming winds.

THE FLORA

On Shasta, the climatic effects of increasing elevation are so significant that the character of the flora changes completely with elevation. Because Mt. Shasta rises as a nearly symmetrical "island" of increasing altitude, an overly simple model of its ecology would depict concentric rings of different floral groupings circling the mountain each at its favored elevation. Of course, such variables as species' different tolerances and the complex effects of slope aspect and drainage make such a model only modestly accurate, but the concept is instructive. In fact, it was on Mt. Shasta that the pioneer ecologist C. Hart Merriam solidified the notion that a higher altitude presents an environment and biota analogous to a higher latitude. A thousand feet of altitude roughly corresponds to about 150 miles of latitude.

Low on Shasta, up to 5500 feet or so, plants find hot, dry summers and cool, rainy winters. Most of these lower slopes are covered with chaparral, dominated by greenleaf manzanita and tobacco brush, a ceanothus. Other chaparral shrubs include oak-like chinquapin, buck-brush ceanothus, antelope brush and Western chokecherry. From a distance the chaparral appears as a pleasant green rug reaching up the mountain, and throughout spring and summer the shrubs erupt with a plethora of flowers and the buzzing of nectar-drunk bees. Among the shrubs grow gardens of flowering herbs, including penstemons, gilia, and the queen of Shasta's flowers, the endangered Shasta lily.

The riot of chaparral growth did not cover the area without help, however. It has taken over since loggers cleared the native forests. In 1898 Merriam wrote, "Shasta rises from a forested region and the mountain itself is continuously forest-covered up to an altitude of 7500 feet or 8000 feet." Photographs and other accounts show that the logging actually started before Merriam's studies, but whenever it started, these native woods were dominated by

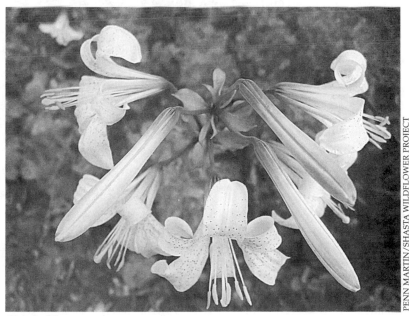

Shasta lily

147

ponderosa pine on the lower slopes and white fir higher up. The chaparral no doubt grew in scattered clearings, and after the logging, the aggressive, sun-loving brush took over.

The chaparral is now very dense, and the shrubs' shade hinders their own seedlings. Pine seedlings, however, need shade, so in theory the forest will eventually overcome the chaparral—assuming no fires or other new disturbances. Since the Great Depression the Forest Service has been planting orderly rows of hybridized ponderosa pine among Shasta's chaparral, in an effort to speed the return of marketable timber.

Above 5500 feet, cooler temperatures, heavier precipitation, and greater distance from logging mills allow conifers to gradually become dominant. Towering over the shrubs you see the long-needled branches of ponderosa pine, the "Christmas tree" spires of white fir and Douglas-fir, the splayed branches of sugar pine and the cone rosettes of knobcone pine. This forest community grows richest on Shasta's southern slopes; sparser trees and more brush characterize the drier northwest wide. On the northeast side, a rather forest of lodgepole pines struggles with the Great Basin influence of cold, dry winters.

Above 6000 feet, almost all precipitation comes as winter snow. Here, one majestic species of tree, Shasta red fir, dominates. Closely related to the red fir of the Sierra, and to noble fir, the Shasta red fir grows mostly farther north in the Cascades. Like its cousins, it has curved combs of blue-green needles, and furrowed maroon bark over a stolid, unbranched trunk. However, unlike red fir proper, Shasta red fir has cones with pointed, papery bracts hanging from each seed envelope; its needles and bark differ subtly from those of noble fir.

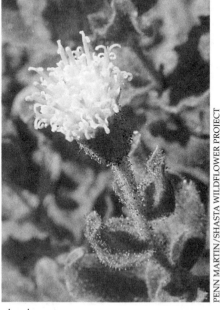

PENN MARTIN/SHASTA WILDFLOWER PROJECT

Arnica

In its other habitats, Shasta red fir grows with one of these cousins, but on Mt. Shasta it rings the mountain in an essentially exclusive forest between 6500 feet and 8000 feet. Another curiosity of Shasta red fir is that to the south it isn't found for 300 miles, until you reach the southern Sierra. This disjointed distribution probably dates from the glacial epochs, when glaciers and a snowy climate likely eliminated the Shasta red fir from most of the Sierra.

Mt. Shasta's porous, dry soils force the firs to keep their distance from one another, so these montane forests of Shasta offer wonderfully open walking and skiing. In the dry duff you notice scattered herbs like white-veined wild ginger, mountain violet and the delicate pink steer's head. In recent decades logging has eaten into the Shasta red-fir forest, leaving precious little forest.

Almost synonymous with the snowy Cascades is the delicate nodding tip of the mountain hemlock, and moist pockets in Shasta's montane forests do foster this graceful tree. In upper Squaw Valley diminutive hemlocks dominate; just above, on the east slopes of Gray Butte, some tall, stout hemlocks compare in stature with red firs. Isolated groves and individuals of mountain hemlock surprise one throughout the montane forests, and up to timberline at 8500 feet.

It's in the openings in the montane forest that the aridity of Shasta's soils is most obvious. At these snowy elevations elsewhere in California and Oregon you'd expect to see green carpets of sedges, grasses and wildflowers, but on Shasta the meadows are sandy—although certainly not without their own floral beauty. Generally one of two flower shrubs dominates, either silver lupine with its purple flower-spikes, or Bloomer's goldenbush with its haphazard, thin yellow petals. Pennyroyal usually wafts its mint-resins through these clearings, and even a casual overview finds paintbrush, phlox, mountain buckwheat, arnica or pussy paws adding summer color between the two dominant shrubs.

Shasta's dry clearings host a few fairly rare plants. Shasta arnica grows only in the Shasta and Crater Lake areas, and Shasta knotweed grows only a little more widely, as far as the northern Sierra. *Phacelia cookei*, a member of the waterleaf family named after Shasta's premier botanist, Dr. William Bridge Cook, grows only on the lower north slopes of Mt. Shasta. The floral relationships of these plants suggest that they have evolved in recent millennia in response to the sandy, dry conditions.

Lusher meadows are found on Shasta, almost exclusively along the profuse springs of Panther and Squaw Valley creeks. Sogginess from these springs keeps the forest at bay, while rushes, sedges and mountain heather flourish. One rare plant, Shasta bluebell, grows only at the springs at the head of Panther Creek and in the Trinity Alps.

Above about 8000, feet red firs and other montane vegetation diminish rapidly. Here you come to timberline, that magical place where only the most ascetic trees live a tenuous existence facing bitter cold, biting winds, late-lying snow, and intense radiation. Although occasional Shasta red firs and mountain hemlocks find niches near timberline, the timberline tree on Shasta is *the* whitebark pine.

The cold winters and late-lying snows on Shasta's north and east slopes offer whitebarks ideal conditions, for here the tree even forms extensive "parkland" forests with many individuals reaching 30-60 feet tall, and scattered specimens that rival the largest whitebarks ever measured. It appears that the whitebarks do so well here partly because on Shasta's colder north and east sides the red firs reach only to about 7500 feet, leaving the pines more lenient habitat. But even the proudest whitebarks reach skyward with twisted and wretched limbs, the naked and bleached relics of growth given up to the elements. It seems that whitebark pines

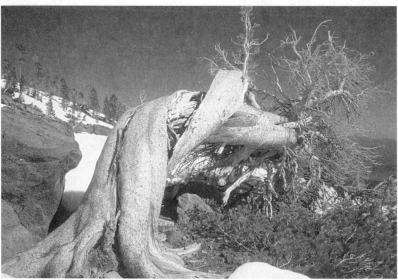

Whitebark pine that has been downed by wind

aren't exactly *adapted* to high mountain environments—they're just more enduring.

Higher than about 8500 feet the whitebarks are dwarfed, huddling close together in thickets often no more than a couple of feet high. Curiously, these *krummholz* ("twisted wood") thickets grow highest along Shasta's exposed ridgecrests, up to 9500 feet, where winter snows melt early and allow a long growing season. The risk of such exposed perches is that winters with little snow leave the needles open to icy, blasting winds; after the 1987-88 drought winter, many timberline whitebarks on Shasta showed extensive die-back.

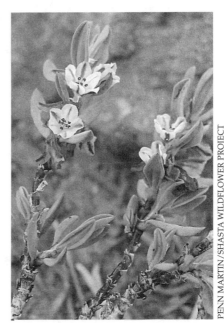

Shasta knotweed

PENN MARTIN/SHASTA WILDFLOWER PROJECT

Growing among the whitebarks, and to even higher elevations, are some perennial wildflowers. These hardy plants are more fully adapted to the alpine life, sucking moisture from the stony earth that to most plants has long since dried up. Although porous Shasta never allows luxuriant alpine growth, Gray's campion, alpine buckwheat, Shasta knotweed, spreading phlox, Lyall's lupine and others splash color across high, sandy slopes. Probably the most ubiquitous flower is the showy white windflower, which nods over ash and talus fields alike. Talus also shelters "softer" plants like mountain heather, alpine sorrel and timberline phacelia.

The toughest of all Shasta's high flowers is Jacob's ladder, a rather tender-looking herb whose snow-white blossoms reportedly grow in lonely rock crevices over 13,000 feet. Its vermiform (wormlike) leaves are thick, spongy and finely hairy to store nutrients and retain water.

Life on Shasta has gone to almost miraculous lengths in even more extreme environments. Colorful lichens crust over rocks nearly to the summit. In summer you might notice a pink tint to the snow, conferred by *Chlamydomonas nivalis*, snow algae. Incredibly, another alga has been identified right in the mud of Shasta's summit hot springs. Withstanding temperatures up to 135°F and an acidity (pH of 1) as strong as battery acid, *Cyanidium caldarium* somehow sustains itself in the fumarole on moisture, minerals and sunlight.

THE FAUNA

BIRDS

Birdwatchers may spy up to 100 species of birds on Mt. Shasta, some living year-round on the mountain, some spending springs and summers here to nest, and some just passing through. Here we introduce the most commonly seen species.

During spring and summer the chaparral practically explodes with avian life, songbirds darting all the daylight hours to feed on the abundant seeds, nectar and insects. You're most likely to see sparrows, warblers, towhees, bluebirds, solitaires and flycatchers—here to breed and rear young, to alight on branches and proclaim territory, bringing a trilling cacophony to Shasta's lower slopes.

In the forests, by comparison, the (merely) numerous birds seem to call down quiet hallways between the big trees. Most commonly one hears the ringing twitters or (in spring) the winsome mating whistles of the mountain chickadee. This bandit-faced bird gleans insects from red-fir boughs. Other calls echoing through the fir forests include the nasal "tin horn" notes of red-breasted nuthatches, the long warbled songs of various Empidonax flycatchers, and the screeches and cries of two bold cousins, the Steller's jay and the gray jay. Woodpeckers drum on the firs, both to announce territory and to drill for insects. Most commonly one sees hairy woodpeckers and white-headed woodpeckers. Nightfall in the forest often brings the haunting calls of a great horned owl.

Among the whitebark pines, Clark's nutcrackers seem to dominate, probably due as much to their loud, brash demeanor as to their sheer numbers. Another jay relative, the Clark's nutcracker gathers whitebark-pine nuts, eating some off the trees and storing many for later.

If you wear red in open areas, you'll likely attract humming-birds, who hope you're a floral nectar source. Both Anna's and rufous hummingbirds make summer stopovers on Shasta to gath-er nectar before returning in late summer to tropical climes.

Raptors occasionally soar over Shasta, scanning the slopes for rodents and reptiles. Most commonly a binocular fix will show the raptor to be a red-tailed hawk, although golden eagles range over the mountain as well, especially over the eastern slopes. A smaller, fast-flying raptor will probably be either a Cooper's hawk or a sharp-shinned hawk.

The lively little birds of Shasta's alpine slopes are finches. Rosy finches (gray-crowned variety) roam to any elevations they please, scooping insects from the glaciers and often chirping to climbers. Mt. Shasta is California's only known nesting site for the coastal Hepburn's rosy finch. Cassin's finches also twitter around tree line and above, snagging bugs off whitebarks.

MAMMALS

Although encounters with mammals on Shasta are rather rare, numerous signs like tracks, scats, burrows and middens hint that mammals are common. Most common are the small herbivores, the rodents that feed on seeds, stems and leaves.

The dainty chipmunks have black and white "racing strips" running down their backs and across their eyes. Most chipmunks on Shasta are yellow-pine chipmunks. They share the chaparral and forests up to about 7000 feet with a similarly striped "squir-rel," the golden-mantled ground squirrel. This animal lacks the stripes on its face, and its plumper build shows that it stores fat for winter hibernation. The slender chipmunk, on the other hand, stores a cache of food to fuel its activities during winter's warm spells.

Shasta's common tree squirrel is the lively Douglas squirrel. One never goes far in the red-fir groves without hearing this rusty-olive animal's long, shrilling calls, or its comical *phews* that punc-tuate its every movement. Shasta is also home to northern flying squirrels, although very few people witness this animal's night-time glides from tree to tree.

You might flush one of two rabbit species on Shasta. If the ears are particularly long, it is a black-tailed hare; if not, a snowshoe hare. Black-tailed hares tend to live below 7000 feet, while snow-shoe hares can be seen up in the whitebark's territory.

The best-known large herbivore on Shasta is the black-tailed deer. These animals migrate between the chaparral and forest zones with the seasons. They especially enjoy new growth, which emerges progressively up the mountain during spring, notably ceanothus leaves and new fir needles.

Canadian elk used to roam on Mt. Shasta, but Muir wrote that by the early 1900s this animal had been hunted from the mountain. However, a herd based down the Sacramento River Canyon at times ranges into Shasta's lower forests.

PREDATORS

Coyotes, foxes, and badgers all feed on squirrels, mice, chipmunks and gophers. Coyotes range all over Shasta, even up to the whitebarks. The gray fox tends to stay in the mid-elevation forests and the chaparral, mixing a diet of rodents with manzanita berries. The red fox is a larger animal that roams subalpine areas, usually meadows. In years past red foxes were seen around Squaw Valley and Panther Meadow, but it may be that increasing numbers of people visiting these meadows have driven them away.

Badgers are low-slung, powerful animals that root out rodents from underground. A burrow on Shasta anywhere below 7500 feet and about 8 inches in diameter will likely be the home of a badger. The marten, a relative of the badger, is a tan-colored tree climber the size of a small dog that snags its prey by sheer guile and quickness. Although extremely rare, the wolverine, a larger, ferocious relative of the badger, may still inhabit the more remote timberline areas of Shasta.

The mountain lion is also quite wary of people, but it undoubtedly still hunts on Shasta, for the authors have seen tracks on Shasta's north flanks. Mountain lions prey chiefly on deer, and they no doubt move up and down the mountain with their prey. Black bears also live on Shasta, in the chaparral and forest zones. These animals are known to eat just about anything, but thankfully on Shasta they have not yet taken to raiding people's stores; the authors know of no instance on Shasta of bears getting into hikers' supplies.

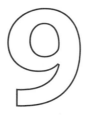

GEOLOGY

MOST OF US RECOGNIZE that Mt. Shasta is a volcano, a "fire mountain" built by eruptions of seething hot rock from the interior of the earth. Indeed, Shasta is one of the largest of the many scores of volcanoes that ring the entire Pacific basin. These volcanoes are a result of the Pacific sea floor spreading east and west. At its margins the sea floor is forced to dive under the adjacent continents and into the earth's hot interior, where it melts. Part of this molten material works up to the surface to erupt and build a volcano.

The earliest eruptions in the Shasta area built the innocuous rise of Everitt Hill, just south of Shasta, about 500,000 years ago. Eruptions that formed Mt. Shasta proper started between 400,000 and 300,000 years ago. In geologic history this is quite recent, and the land that Shasta grew upon no doubt closely resembled its surroundings today.

By 300-250,000 years ago there stood an early Mt. Shasta perhaps about as high as the present peak. We know very little about this proto-Shasta, for only a spiny, eroded segment remains of its original cone. This remnant forms the southeast side of Shasta, from Clear Creek to the east rim of Avalanche Gulch.

About 30,000 years ago eruptions started to stack up a new cone, northwest of the original cone. Material from the new vent became what is now Casaval Ridge and most of the eastern flank of Shasta. A later eruption of this vent built up Misery Hill, the dark bane of climbers nearing the top of Shasta's most popular climbing route. About 9500 years ago this vent's final gasp spilled forth the Red Banks, the brow of welded pumice that caps Avalanche Gulch.

About this same time, 10-9000 years ago, the vent that rapidly built Shastina opened up. Soon after, subsidiary vents on young Shastina's north flank poured forth lava flows that still look fresh

155

today. Northeast of Weed, Hwy. 97 takes a curving detour around the bluff of what locals call "Lava Park."

Another striking feature of Shastina is the deep gash in its west face—Diller Canyon. Geologists aren't sure whether an inward collapse or an outward blast initiated this huge ravine, but in any case as Shastina grew it sent repeated eruptions of superheated rocks (pyroclastic flows) down it, scouring out the gulch and deeply burying the site of present-day Weed.

Shasta's most recent eruptions have stacked up a fourth cone, which makes up most of Shasta's northern flank and the summit area. One impressive legacy of this most recent vent is the Military Pass lava flow. Striking today even on a topo map, this flow poured down the canyon of Inconstance Creek to about 6100 feet, several thousand years ago. This vent continued erupting until just a few hundred years ago, and as testimony that it's not necessarily finished, a couple of small hot springs just west of Shasta's highest crags still hiss and bubble with sulfurous gases and water.

Like the eruptions of all the other Cascade volcanoes, Shasta's have varied in character, spewing out gas, molten lava, semi-molten rocks, cinders (small particles) and ash (very fine particles) in various proportions. The products of the different eruptions cool to form different layers, or strata, of rock types, so Shasta is a *stratovolcano*. The major types of strata are lava and tuff. Lava is formed by a flow that is fluid and coherent, that spreads rather broadly, and that when cool forms blocky, fairly solid rock. Tuff results from semi–molten ejected materials that settle together and congeal, often forming unstable cliffs. It's the interlayering of tuffs and lavas over the course of many eruptions that allows stratovolcanoes to stand so tall: tuff layers steepen the slopes and lava layers provide strength.

However, as one geologist put it, "Volcanoes can be thought of as ephemeral aggregations of unstable material." Studies of Shasta Valley, just northwest of Mt. Shasta, show just how unstable a volcano can be. Scores of hillocks and mounds pimple the terrain here; geologists now realize that these are eroded blocks of debris from a monstrous landslide off of the old proto-Mt. Shasta—the largest known landslide in the last million years. About 360-300,000 years ago an estimated 26 cubic kilometers sloughed off the mountain, ran down the Shasta River plain past the present site of Yreka, and temporarily choked off the Klamath River. Although an earthquake or an eruption might have triggered the cataclysm, no evidence suggests this. The collapse may have been simply the fall of an oversteepened slope.

Smaller cataclysms have resulted when Shasta has erupted and melted glaciers and snow, as it often has. For instance, about 3000 years ago eruption-caused floods ran down Mud Creek Canyon, and the debris now underlies the town of McCloud and much of lower Squaw Valley beyond.

NEIGHBORING CONES

Even a brief drive through the Shasta area reveals other volcanic vents. Most obvious is Black Butte, about 9500 years old, a steep cone that rises some 2400 feet above adjacent I-5. Another, older cone is Ash Creek Butte, 9 miles east-northeast of Mt. Shasta. Aligning more or less north and south of Shasta are the smaller buttes near North Gate, Red Butte, Gray Butte, McKenzie Butte and its satellites, and Everitt Hill. This pattern suggests an underlying north-south weakness in the earth's crust here.

SHASTA'S GLACIERS

Glaciers form on high, cold mountains, where more snow accumulates during the winter than can melt during the summer. Over the decades the "excess" snow piles up and gradually compacts into ice. Eventually it gains enough weight to start creeping and flowing downhill. This river of ice rides down with almost irresistible force, pushing aside and grinding down rocks. Eventually the glacier's front reaches lower elevations where warmer climes melt it away. In this way a glacier is a gravity-driven system that dissipates "excess" snowfall.

Glaciers wax and wane with changes in the climate, and a persistent cooling of just a few degrees will bring on a glacial era. In a snowy but relatively warm climate like Shasta's, it is thought that cooler, cloudier summers are especially needed for glacier formation. When Shasta first formed, the northern hemisphere seems to have had such conditions, so glaciers have no doubt periodically draped the mountain virtually since its inception.

Geologists can estimate the previous extent of glaciers partly by the characteristic mounds of debris, called moraines, that the ice rivers leave behind. The presence of moraines around Shasta may be evidence that during at least one glacial period, ice from the south slopes of Shasta merged with ice from Mt. Eddy. This ice then flowed to near the present site of Dunsmuir, to the north glaciers pooled in Shasta Valley, and to the east where Shasta's ice probably joined with glaciers from the Medicine Lake highlands.

The climate around Shasta has not always supported glaciers, however. At about the same time that Shastina was forming, a warm and dry period melted all permanent ice on the mountain. From 9000 to 3000 years ago, geologists think there were at least a couple of glacial advances, but for much of this period Shasta probably held little or no ice. Starting about 3000 years ago, a cooler and wetter period brought on the "Little Ice Age," and fairly extensive glaciers accumulated on the mountain, probably even on its sunnier south slopes. This "neo-glaciation" continued strong into the late 1700s, and Shasta's present glaciers persist on a reduced scale from this time.

Today at least eight distinct glaciers flow down Mt. Shasta, including by far the largest ones in California. The Whitney Glacier is largest of all, pouring down between Shasta and Shastina, carting away debris from the flanks of both peaks. The Whitney shows multiple crevasses, long cracks that formed when terrain underneath distorted the glacier's flow and generated tension in it. Snow can bridge these slots, sometimes thickly enough to obscure the gap but too thin to hold a climber's weight. To help keep from falling into these insidious traps, on snow-covered glaciers climbers use roped travel. The Whitney Glacier also spills over a couple of very steep sections, where the ice fractures into blocky, spectacular icefalls.

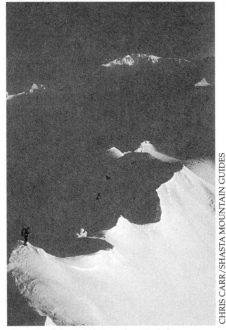

CHRIS CARR/SHASTA MOUNTAIN GUIDES

Overlooking Avalanche Gulch

Shasta's second largest glacier (in volume) is the Hotlum, which flows northeast from near the summit. The Hotlum also breaks into

158

two or three icefalls. Relatively dry years since the 1920s have isolated a lobe of the Hotlum, and this has become known as the Chicago Glacier, for the annual studies conducted here by the University of Chicago.

The Wintun Glacier has a fairly active core section, which forms a small icefall as it drops into Ash Creek's upper canyon. The Bolam Glacier is extensive too, but its few crevasses and its gently sloping, receding terminus shows that it is relatively inactive.

Shasta's three other glaciers flow out of small, sheltered cirques in the mountain's southeast headwalls. The Konwakiton and Mud Creek glaciers (the latter is also called the Stuhl Glacier) spill out of small basins above Mud Creek; the Konwakiton is especially active and fractured for its small size. The recently recognized Watkins Glacier commemorates amateur geologist R.H. Watkins, who described this glacier and the post-1940 rejuvenation of Shasta's glaciers in general long before "official" geologists took notice.

The "neo-glaciation" gradually waned during the 19th century. At the turn of the century Shasta's glaciers briefly resurged, but soon after that a few warm, dry decades dramatically diminished them. The Wintun especially dwindled to just a vestige of stagnant ice. It wasn't until the 1940s that heavier snowfalls returned and rejuvenated the glaciers; for instance, by 1972 the Whitney had extended more than 1500 feet beyond its withered position of 1944. (Climatologists believe that the next few decades will be warmer and probably drier. And in the longer term the "greenhouse effect" will probably bring even drier and warmer conditions.)

The wild fluctuations of northern California's climate in the last two decades have brought visible changes to Shasta's glaciers. The record winters of 1982 and 1983 started a "wave" of thicker ice moving down their lengths. Then the warmth of the drought years of 1986-92 melted away those gains. No new snow accumulated, leaving very icy conditions for climbers on the north-side routes. The Bolam and Wintun glaciers, especially, began to thin appreciably. Then very heavy and late winters again in the late 1990s started another wave of thickening ice.

Hot summers occasionally cause Shasta's glaciers to release outburst floods called *jokulhlaups*. This happens when melt water somehow pools up in a glacier, then bursts free. In 1924 Shasta's most infamous jokulhlaups gushed out of either the Konwakiton or the Mud Creek glacier, collected ice, mud and rocks on its way down between Mud Creek's unstable canyon walls, then rumbled beyond the mountain and damaged structures in McCloud. Silt from the flood choked off fish in the McCloud River and, some say, even clouded San Francisco Bay. Smaller outburst floods have raced down most of Shasta's canyons in this century—typically about once every 10 years—including some from the Whitney Glacier that in 1985 and 1998 covered Hwy. 97 and threatened homes to the north.

What everyone would like to know, of course, is, "Will Mt. Shasta erupt again, and if so, when?" The geologic record gives every reason to believe that Mt. Shasta will erupt again, potentially destroying nearby towns. Imminent eruptions usually give enough warning for people to evacuate, but no one can now predict when such a future eruption might occur. During the last few millennia Mt. Shasta has erupted on the average every 250-300 years, and the last small eruption may have occurred in 1786, when la Perouse apparently saw signs of one from his ship off the coast. From the late summer of 1978 through January 1981 periodic swarms of minor earthquakes shook the area, mostly centered east of Ash Creek Butte. These earthquakes were exactly the sort that indicate rising magma, but since then there has been only quiet.

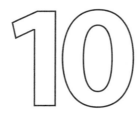

AMENITIES, SOURCES,
AND OTHER INFORMATION

VISITOR INFORMATION

The towns at the foot of Mt. Shasta have a full range of supplies, services, food and lodging. You can obtain brochures and other useful information by writing or calling the Chamber of Commerce office in each town:

Mount Shasta: 300 Pine Street, Mount Shasta, CA 96067, (800) 926-4865, (530) 926-4865; www.mtshastachamber.com

McCloud: P.O. Box 372, McCloud, CA 96057, (530) 964-3113

Dunsmuir 4841 Dunsmuir Ave., Dunsmuir, CA 96025, (530) 235-2177

Weed: P.O. Box 366, Weed, CA 96094, (530) 938-4624

Siskiyou County Visitors Bureau: P.O. Box 1138, Mount Shasta, CA 96067, (530) 926-3850; www.visitsiskiyou.org, www.visitmtshasta.org

Mt. Shasta is located within the Shasta–Trinity National Forest. The Forest Supervisor's office is at 2400 Washington Ave., Redding, CA 96001, (530) 244-2978. There are two district ranger offices in charge of the Shasta area, one in Mount Shasta and one in McCloud. Wilderness, climbing, and campfire permits, trail guides, campground information, and various informative brochures are available at the offices. The Mt. Shasta Ranger District office maintains a complete visitor information facility. They also have an interpretive association retail outlet for a wide selection of books, maps, guides and even video tapes. A mail-order catalog is also available.

Mt. Shasta Ranger District
204 West Alma Street
Mount Shasta, CA 96067
(530) 926-4511
Recorded recreational information: (530) 926-9613
Weather and climbing information:
www.shastaavalanche.org

Office hours: Winter (November through April),
Monday-Friday, 8:00 a.m.–4:30 p.m.; Summer (May
through Oct.),
7 days per week 8:00-4:30

McCloud Ranger District
Minnesota Ave. and Hwy. 89
McCloud, CA 96057
(530) 964-2184
Office hours: Winter (November through April),
Monday-Friday, 8:00 a.m.–4:30 p.m.; Summer (May
through Oct.), 7 days per week 8:00-4:30

The **Mt. Shasta Ranger District** maintains the following campgrounds:

Castle Lake: 11.5 miles southwest of Mount Shasta on Castle Lake road.

Gumboot: 15 miles southwest of Mount Shasta on South Fork road.

McBride Springs: 4.5 miles northeast of Mount Shasta on Everitt Memorial Highway.

Panther Meadow: 13.5 miles northeast of Mount Shasta on Everitt Memorial Highway.

Toad Lake: 18 miles west of Mount Shasta off South Fork road, via Morgan Meadow road.

The **McCloud Ranger District** maintains the following campgrounds:

Ah-Di-Na: 4 miles south of Lake McCloud off Hwy 89.

Algoma: 14 miles east of McCloud off Hwy. 89.

Cattle Camp: 11 miles east of McCloud off Hwy. 89.

Fowler's Camp: 6.5 miles east of McCloud off Hwy. 89.

Harris Springs: 17 miles north of Bartle off Hwy. 89.

Trout Creek: 20 miles northeast of McCloud on Pilgrim Creek road, off Hwy. 89.

Other campgrounds include:

Castle Crags State Park
Castella, CA 96017
(530) 235-2684

There are two privately owned campgrounds both of which have excellent facilities. Lake Siskiyou Campground is located 3 miles west of Mount Shasta on the South Fork road. There are 299 campsites, and you'll also find showers, a store, a marina and a beach. There's excellent swimming in the lake, as well as boating, fishing and windsurfing.

Lake Siskiyou Campground
P.O. Box 276
Mount Shasta, CA 96067
(530) 926-2618
www.lakesis.com

A spacious KOA campground is conveniently located at the north end of Mount Shasta City. There are 110 campsites and complete facilities.

KOA Campground
900 N. Mt. Shasta Blvd.
Mount Shasta, CA 96067
(530) 926-4029

DRIVING TOURS

The ranger offices have many free maps and information on driving tours to points of interest in the area. Two of the best trips are: Around Mt. Shasta via Military Pass Road, and the Seven Lakes Basin loop tour. Plan on a full day for each of these scenic jaunts.

MUSEUMS

The Sisson Museum, located on the grounds of the Mt. Shasta Fish Hatchery, is open year-round. Operated entirely by volunteers, the museum has many permanent displays on the history of Siskiyou County—particularly Mt. Shasta—as well as temporary shows that change several times a year. The hatchery itself is the oldest one in California. You will enjoy seeing the giant, docile brood trout swimming in their pools.

Sisson Museum

Hatchery Lane and Old Stage Rd. (off Central I-5 exit), Mount Shasta

(530) 926-5508: hours 10 a.m.–5 p.m. daily.

www.mountshastasissonmuseum.org

The College of the Siskiyous Library in Weed has one of the most extensive special collections of books, manuscripts, photographs, and rare materials all pertaining to Mt. Shasta.

College of the Siskiyous

800 College Avenue, Weed

(530) 938-5331; hours by appointment

for special collection.

www.siskiyous.edu/library/shasta/html

RECREATION

Shops in Mount Shasta that carry and rent outdoor equipment. (All addresses are: Mount Shasta, CA 96067, unless otherwise indicated)

The Fifth Season

426 N. Mt. Shasta Blvd.

(530) 926-3606

www.thefifthseason.com

The Fifth Season also has a 24-hour recorded phone message for the latest climbing and skiing conditions on the mountain: (530) 926-5555.

The House of Ski & Board

316 Chestnut Street

(530) 926-2359

www.shastaski.com

The two above also rent ice axes, crampons and boots for climbing. Reserve in advance for holiday weekends.

The Sportsmen's Den
402 N. Mt. Shasta Blvd.
(530) 926-2295

GUIDE SERVICE

There are several professional guides and outfitters in the Shasta area who operate under permit from the U.S. Forest Service. Their activities include mountain climbing, ski touring, river rafting, fishing, pack trips and more. Several offer specialized trips for families, kids, and the physically disabled. You can obtain current listings of these outfitters, as well as brochures and information, from the district ranger offices.

Shasta Mountain Guides
PO Box 1543
(530) 926-3117
www.shastaguides.com

WHITEWATER RAFTING AND KAYAKING

Living Waters Recreation
PO Box 1192
(530) 926-5446, (800) 994-7238
www.livingwatersrec.com

River Dancers
302 Terry Lynn
(530) 926-3517, (800) 926-5002
www.riverdancers.com

Turtle River Rafting Co.
PO Box 313
(530) 926-3223, (800 726-3223
www.turtleriver.com

Osprey Outdoors Kayak School
2925 Cantara Rd.
(530) 926-6310
www.ospreykayak.com

FISHING GUIDES

Jack Trout Guide Service
PO Box 94
(530) 926-4540
www.jacktrout.com

Craig Nielsen – Shasta Trout
512 Sarah Bell
(530) 926-5763
www.shastatrout.com

Alan Blankenship
16725 Friar Pl.
Weed, CA 96094
(530) 938-1514
www.threeriversguideservice.com

Ron Hart Guide Service
965 Lassen Lane
(530) 926-2482
Rick Cox Guide Service
(530) 964-2533

DOWNHILL SKIING

The **Mt. Shasta Board & Ski Park** is 10 miles from I-5 via Hwy. 89.

Office: 104 Siskiyou Ave.
(800) 754-7427; (530) 926-8610;
Snowphone: (530) 926-8686
www.skipark.com

SNOW PLAY AREA

The Forest Service maintains a snow play area for sledding and sliding at **Snowman's Hill**, 6 miles east of I-5 on Hwy. 89.

OTHER REFERENCES

Mt. Shasta Trail Association
PO Box 36
Mount Shasta, CA 96067

The Mt. Shasta Trail Association is a nonprofit public benefit organization whose purpose is to design, construct, maintain, and use trails in the Mt. Shasta area. The public is invited to participate in various trail projects, as well as scheduled hiking, canoeing, birding, and bicycling trips.

The Sierra Club Foundation Shasta Alpine Lodge
The Foundation cabin at Horse Camp on Mt. Shasta has an informative website and links:
www.tscf.org/foundation/horse_camp

Pacific Crest Trail Association
www.pcta.org
The PCTA maintains and preserves the Pacific Crest Trail, including portions of the trail in the region of Mt. Shasta.

California Wilderness Coalition
www.calwild.org
The CWC is a non-profit organization dedicated to preserving and enhancing California wilderness.

Upper Sacramento River Exchange
PO Box 784
Dunsmuir, CA 96025
(530) 235-2012

The River Exchange promotes healthy watersheds through stewardship, education, restoration, and community involvement.
www.riverexchange.org

Shasta Wildflower Project
P.O. Box 583
Mount Shasta, CA 96067
(530) 926-3398

Interpretive hikes on and around Mt. Shasta to some of the area's most spectacular wildflower habitats.
www.shastawildflowers.com

The Nature Conservancy McCloud River Preserve
(530) 926-4366
www.nature.org

Stewardship Fund of Far Northern California
PO Box 1586
Mount Shasta, CA 96067
(530) 926-6670

Caring for natural, historical, and rural surroundings throughout northern California.
www.e-jedi.org/travelgreen

Siskiyou Land Trust
PO Box 183
Mount Shasta, CA 96067
(530) 926-2259

Promoting long-term land stewardship in Siskiyou County
www.siskiyoulandtrust.org

USEFUL INFORMATION

EMERGENCY

Fire, police, ambulance, highway patrol: Dial **911**.

TRANSPORTATION

The closest passenger air service to Mt. Shasta is Redding, CA and Medford, OR.

Amtrak: 24-hour information: (800) USA-RAIL

Holiday Travel Bureau
319 N. Mt. Shasta Blvd.
(877) 926-3491, (530) 926-3491

Eagle Nest Aviation
Scenic flights and charter service
PO Box 241, Gazelle, CA 96034
(530) 938-2656

ROAD AND WEATHER

National Weather Service, 24-hour recorded message: (530) 221-5613

California Highway Patrol, 24-hour report on road conditions: (530) 842-2716

www.wunderground.com (click on: Mt. Shasta, CA)
www.weather.com (click on: Mt. Shasta, CA)
www.avalanche.org (click on: Mt. Shasta, CA)

SELF-SERVICE WILDERNESS PERMITS

Self-service permits can be issued at the following trailheads on Mt. Shasta: Bunny Flat, North Gate, Clear Creek, and Brewer Creek.

AFTERWORD

WE'RE ALL GUESTS, caretakers and cohabitants of this planet. In the 21st century environmental concern—and environmental degradation—have reached global proportions. Mt. Shasta, like many other unique micro-environments, shows man's impact.

Some common-sense guidelines apply to Mt. Shasta, as well as other wilderness areas:

• Be a thoughtful backcountry visitor. Know something about your route and the area, and follow the management guidelines of the governing agencies.

• Accept the responsibility of knowing the basics of first aid, navigation and minimum-impact camping.

• Choose your campsites thoughtfully, and leave them in as natural a state as possible. Keep groups small and blend camps and tents into the environment.

• Even where a fire is possible, consider a fireless evening. Wildlands are feeling the effects of too many fires.

• Always use established latrines if they exist. If not, always use human waste pack-out bags.

• Do everything you can to protect water sources from contamination. Although giardia has not yet been reported on Mt. Shasta, its occurrence is increasing in the backcountry generally.

INDEX

MAP INDEX

Aerial Photos

ABOUT THE AUTHORS

Andy Selters, below right, started his climbing career on Mt. Shasta, and he has gone on to guide and climb all over the world, from Alaska to Yosemite, British Columbia to Bolivia, and Washington to Nepal. He has written a variety of other books on hiking and mountaineering and its history. Currently he lives in Bishop, California.

California native **Michael Zanger** has been hooked on the mountains ever since a family trip to Yosemite at the age of five. He founded Shasta Mountain Guides in the mid-1970s, and has lived at the foot of Mt. Shasta for nearly 40 years. In addition to Mt. Shasta, Michael has participated in climbs and expeditions in North and South America, Europe, Africa, and Asia. He is also the author of the book on the history of Mt. Shasta, *Mt. Shasta: History, Legend, and Lore.*

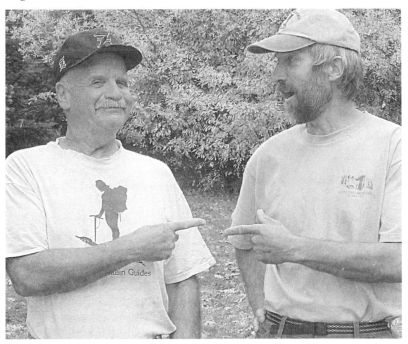

Also available from WILDERNESS PRESS

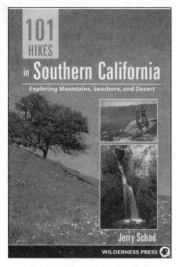

Veteran author Jerry Schad reveals his top picks for the the finest hiking adventures in the Southland. Trek the diverse terrain of Southern California with the ultimate guide to the 101 best hikes, from 1-mile strolls to 20-mile challenges. Covers Santa Monica, San Gabriel, San Jacinto, and San Bernardino mountains, and the Mojave and Colorado deserts.

ISBN 978-0-89997-351-7

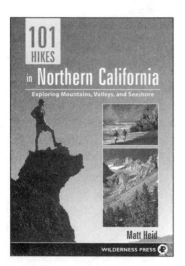

Discover Northern California's finest hiking opportunities, from Big Sur to Sequoia National Park, from the Lost Coast to the Modoc Plateau. You'll find hikes for every season, skill level, and interest. Some hikes are well known, and others are a well-kept secret. Whether you want to take it easy with a 1-mile stroll, or challenge yourself with a 16-mile epic adventure, you'll find a hike that's right for you.

ISBN 978-0-89997-474-3

For ordering information, contact your local bookseller or Wilderness Press, www.wildernesspress.com.